Health Care of Women:
A Gynecological Assessment

Health Care of Women: A Gynecological Assessment

Joellen Watson Hawkins

Loretta P. Higgins

Wadsworth Health Sciences Division

Monterey, California

Wadsworth Health Sciences Division
A Division of Wadsworth, Inc.

Printed in the United States of America

10 9 8 7 6 5 4 3 2 1

Library of Congress Cataloging in Publication Data

Hawkins, Joellen Watson.
    Health care of women.

    Includes bibliographies and index.
    1. Gynecologic nursing. I. Higgins, Loretta
Pierfedeici. I. Title. (DNLM: 1. Gynecology—Nursing
texts. WY 156.7 H393h)
RG105.H37   618.1′0024613   81–16245
ISBN 0-8185-0505-2   AACR2

Sponsoring Editors: *Edward Murphy/James Keating*
Production: *Ron Newcomer & Associates, San Francisco, California*
Manuscript Editor: *Carol Westberg*
Interior Design: *Jamie Sue Brooks*
Cover Design: *Albert Burkhardt*
Illustrations: *Cyndie Clark-Huegel*
Typesetting: *Computer Typesetting Services, Inc., Glendale, California*

To Andrew, Daniel, David, Glen, John, Karen, Marshall, Terry, and our parents.

Preface

Nurses are beginning to assume more responsibility for primary health care of women in gynecologic settings. As their roles change, they need to expand their knowledge base and skills. This book is designed for use in certificate courses and degree programs that prepare nurses to become gynecologic nurse practitioners.

Many nurses who are primary care providers for women spend a great deal of their time in assessment, primary prevention, and health teaching. This book is intended as a supplement and complement to basic textbooks concerned with gynecologic nursing, women's health, physical assessment, and gynecology. Its focus is on primary prevention and health maintenance.

This text is designed to: (1) provide materials on health assessment of women, (2) discuss normal findings and common aberrations, and (3) present information on primary prevention and nursing interventions for common acute, self-limiting, episodic problems. It can be used with nursing process and POMR (problem-oriented medical record format). All case studies and client names are fictitious.

Behavioral Objectives

At the completion of this book, the learner should be able to:

1. describe and analyze the interview components of a gynecologic examination
2. identify and describe the anatomy and physiology of the woman's reproductive tract and breasts

3. evaluate equipment necessary for the examination and for laboratory specimens
4. analyze the steps of the external and internal gynecologic examination
5. evaluate common findings and their probable causes and significance
6. correlate findings with appropriate nursing interventions
7. evaluate need for medical referral
8. analyze the steps of examination, self-breast exam (SBE), and findings
9. analyze components of health care for women that are of special concern for providers
10. synthesize and write up findings from the interview and physical assessment components of the gynecologic examination.

The authors wish to acknowledge the support and encouragement of their colleagues and students during this project, especially of the nurse practitioners, staff, and nursing director of the Women's Health Clinic, Student Health Services, University of Connecticut. To our loyal typists, Carol Kozak and Janice Bittner, we can never say an adequate thank you. We are especially grateful to Ed Murphy and Jim Keating, our editors, for their support and faith in us. To those closest to us, our deepest appreciation for the chores done, errands run, love, and support that made this book possible.

Joellen Watson Hawkins
Loretta P. Higgins

Contents

Health Care of Women:
A Gynecological Assessment

Introduction to the Gynecologic Examination: Interview Components

At the end of Chapter 1, you will be able to identify, describe, and evaluate the following:

1. the setting for a gynecologic exam
2. interviewing techniques pertinent to the ambulatory gynecologic setting
3. the components of the complete health history
4. the components of a systems review
5. the write-up for the interview portion of the exam

The Setting

The setting for a complete gynecologic examination should offer privacy, an unhurried atmosphere, and an opportunity for the woman and nurse to sit and talk face to face. It should assure the client that she and what she says are important. Nothing is less conducive to sharing important information and developing a sense of trust than lack of privacy or an examination in which all the interviewing takes place with the client undressed and on the examining table. The intimate nature of this examination, the possibility of a need to share information about aspects of sexuality, and societal influences must be acknowledged in providing a setting that will maximize privacy and protect confidentiality.

Interviewing Techniques

Interviewing skills are critical to putting your client at ease and eliciting data necessary for a complete assessment. Data must be relevant to the assessment process. It is important that you, as the interviewer, understand the rationale for the data you are collecting and convey to your client why these data are necessary. Assuring confidentiality and informing the client of her rights concerning information elicited and her medical records should be part of the interview process.

You set the stage for the interview. Introduce yourself to all of your clients. They have a right to know who you are just as you know who they are. A number of behaviors will help you put your client at ease, such as being attentive, making an effort to establish rapport, offering courtesy and respect to your client as a person, providing freedom from interruption (as much as possible), and maintaining a caring objectivity.[1] An atmosphere of acceptance and trust will aid you in eliciting data necessary to a careful, thorough assessment and help the client to perceive you as a caring, supportive health-care provider.

During the interview, observe the nonverbal as well as verbal cues the woman gives you as she enters the examining room or office. Does she appear upset or nervous? Is she wringing her hands, perspiring profusely, or demonstrating by other gestures that she is anxious? Does she make eye contact when speaking with you? Does she sit comfortably in

2

the chair or appear stiff and on edge? If clients fill out a history or information form before you see them, what can you learn from that? Has the woman ever been examined before? Has she had a pelvic examination and a Pap smear? Is she experiencing symptoms that may be perceived as threatening to her body image or integrity or that may cause fear of cancer, infection, venereal disease, or pregnancy? Can you learn anything from basic data such as place of residence, age, culture, or occupation that will help you be sensitive to her needs and concerns?

What does she tell you first? Are answers to questions elaborate or monosyllabic? How would you describe her affect and appearance? Does she express feelings with any display of emotion?

Recognition and acknowledgment of the developmental stage is important in assessing any client. The interview portion of the health assessment will enable you to ascertain the client's developmental stage and correlate it with her chronological age.

Working with adolescents demands recognition of developmental tasks, assurance of confidentiality, and respect for their struggle for independence. Be sensitive to the impatience that is characteristic of adolescence and give feedback, information, and opinions as soon as possible. Prejudgment can cause the care giver to omit pertinent questions. Awareness of biases and stereotypes can enable the health-care provider to remain nonjudgmental and open.[2] If a parent or parents accompany the adolescent, the needs and rights of the adolescent must be respected in a way that will also promote dialogue with parents.

The rights of minors to acquire contraception and to request an abortion are far from clear under the laws of the United States. Decisions made in two cases have resulted in the right of minors to purchase and use contraceptives in spite of parental or state dissent. The Supreme Court has ruled that statutes requiring parental consent for an unmarried minor to have an abortion are unconstitutional.[3] Current legislation and trends, however, challenge this decision. While recognizing that the rights of minors to privacy should be upheld, the court nonetheless suggests that those rights may be more limited than for adults. Some support for the rights of states to assist parents in influencing health-care decisions for their minor children seems evident from court decisions thus far.[3] Complex issues of states' authority to define rights and parental control over health-care decisions of minors are involved. Cases now before the courts will help to carve out the definitions of the health-care rights of minors.[4]

Older persons often have long health histories. The nurse should sit near, maintain eye contact, and be aware of any indication of a limitation such as hearing loss that may impair the interview process.[5] The nature of gynecological care often dictates the need for asking questions that the client may view as embarrassing or personal. Explaining the importance of information to the assessment process and assuring confidentiality may help to put the woman at ease.

History Taking

At the beginning of the interview, some general information about the woman is elicited:

1. age
2. date and place of birth (any complications the client is aware of)
3. marital status (relationships if pertinent)
4. place of residence and conditions (live alone or with others)
5. informant and reliability (self or other)
6. educational level, student status
7. occupation, present employment, past if pertinent, hours of work (nights, evenings)
8. health insurance
9. exercise and activities

If some of this general information is already included in forms the client has filled out, you should not request it again. Be sensitive to this issue as you continue eliciting information.

Cultural history

The meaning and value of reproduction and reproductive organs is very important and pertinent to gynecologic examination and interventions. If the woman is a member of a culture that values reproduction highly and discourages sexual expression except for conception, contraceptives will probably not be acceptable, and any threat, perceived or real, to reproductive integrity will be anxiety-producing. Taboos should be explored. These may include touching one's genital area (precluding use of a diaphragm and perhaps even use of vaginal cream to treat an infection), pelvic examination before marriage, and examination by a male. It is important to clarify and be supportive of any rituals or cultural beliefs surrounding sexuality. To the woman who highly values the "miracle baby" resulting from coitus interruptus, other contraceptive practices may be unacceptable.

Dietary practices may relate to fertility, the menses, and reproductive functioning. Elicit information so that interventions that would interfere with practices will not be planned. A lack of response may not mean agreement, but deference to authority. Clients are often labeled noncompliant when, in fact, they are unwilling to violate cultural beliefs or when they misinterpret the intention of modes of therapy.

Understanding of the meanings of health care, perceptions of what health is, and the concepts of primary prevention will assist the client and provider in reaching an understanding of each one's expectations.

Because a gynecologic examination requires tactile contact of examiner with client, it is also important to know meanings and taboos surrounding touch. Paralinguistic behaviors (tone of voice, pitch and speed of vocalization), kinesic behaviors (facial expression, eye contact, posture, and so on), and proxemic behaviors (spatial relationships) directly affect the client's perceptions of the care provider as caring or threatening.[6] None of this means that the nurse as care provider should divest herself of her own cultural background and influences, but rather that she should be sensitive to, responsive to, and noninterfering with those of her clients.

The cultural history might include components such as:

1. meaning of reproduction
2. attitudes toward sexual expression
3. taboos in relation to touch, to genitals, or to breasts
4. acceptance of gynecological examination, especially by a male or prior to marriage
5. beliefs concerning use of contraception, fertility
6. perceptions of health and health care, value of preventive measures such as immunization and contraception

If a client is seeking care for a specific health problem, the nurse should assess:

1. beliefs about the cause of the problem
2. beliefs about the cure
3. self-medication
4. self-treatment
5. treatment by family
6. treatment by folk practitioners[7]

Family history

In taking a family history as a component of the gynecologic exam, it is especially pertinent to ask about:

1. cardiovascular disease, arteriosclerosis
2. hypertension

3. cancer especially of genital tract and breasts
4. diabetes, adult and juvenile onset
5. hypercholesterolemia
6. reproductive tract or breast problems, especially in sisters or mother
7. varicose veins, phlebitis, clotting disorders
8. migraine headaches
9. allergies
10. cerebral vascular accidents
11. venereal disease
12. spontaneous abortions, pregnancy loss, complications
13. menstrual problems
14. sickle-cell anemia, other blood dyscrasias and hematologic disorders
15. renal disease

Many of these are familial and/or relate to decisions regarding contraception, to general health status, and directly or indirectly to sexuality, the menstrual cycle, and reproductive organs.

Drug history

Information about medications taken regularly and occasionally, including the use of over-the-counter (OTC) drugs and recreational drugs, comprises an important part of the history. Also include use of alcohol (time and number of drinks per day or week) and smoking (number of cigarettes per day, type and duration of habit, any use of marijuana).

Diet history

A diet history and longitudinal survey of weight and height provide useful data for the total profile. When taking a diet history, be specific. Inquire as to the size of servings; whether fruit and vegetables are fresh, frozen, or canned; how food is prepared, whether grain products used are whole grain or processed. Ask about use of condiments and beverages, including sweeteners or dairy products used in them. You should also inquire about typical daily eating patterns including snacks and, if pertinent, where most meals are eaten (home, brown bag, or in a restaurant), who shops, and who plans and prepares food.

Current Complaint

Ask the woman to tell you the reason for the visit. Have her describe her symptoms, their duration, severity, persistence, changes, exacerbation or remissions, how she has coped, and what, if anything, has brought relief. Ask her if she has ever experienced similar symptoms before and, if so, under what circumstances. How long did the symptoms last and what made them disappear or abate?

Systems Review

Reproductive tract

A complete reproductive system review includes the following:

1. menstrual history—onset of puberty, age at menarche, duration of cycles, description of cycles, dysmenorrhea, discomforts and symptoms, signs of ovulation, date of last menstrual period, intermenstrual bleeding, age at menopause, symptoms, postmenopausal bleeding, any use of estrogens postmenopause
2. pregnancies and abortions—duration, symptoms, termination and outcomes, complications, health status of any children
3. DES (diethylstilbestrol) exposure in daughters whose mothers took drugs during pregnancies or a personal history of taking DES during pregnancy or to suppress lactation
4. sexually transmissible (venereal) diseases, genital warts, vaginal infections—type, duration, symptoms, treatment, recurrence
5. date of last Pap smear, results; any abnormal Pap smears ever
6. contraception—types used, satisfaction, problems, side effects, duration of use, present method, any failures; sterilization method and any problems
7. sexual history—libido, responses, dyspareunia, orgasm, problems, any infertility, postcoital bleeding, sexually active at present, trauma (including rape)
8. urinary tract—frequency, burning, urgency, hematuria, incontinence, dysuria, urethritis, irritation around meatus
9. constipation, diarrhea, pain in rectal area
10. hygiene—douching (method, reason, solution), deodorants, tampons, sanitary pads, soaps (laundry products and bath), talcum powder, type of underclothing, use of bubble bath
11. any surgery of reproductive organs (dates and results)—tubal ligation, D & C, hysterectomy, repair of cystocele, rectocele
12. symptoms at present—cystocele, rectocele, stress incontinence, prolapse of uterus, signs of infection (pruritis, type and amount of discharge, irritation, rash), masses, lesions, nodules, tenderness or pain, headache, change in vaginal discharge, odor, enlarged glands or nodes, unusual bleeding, problems with contraception

Breasts and lymphatics

A review of the client's history concerning breasts and lymphatics includes:

1. development—when, normalcy of pattern, any problems
2. discharge (amount and character), lactation (duration, success, supply, problems), any possibility of pregnancy
3. changes in size, pigmentation, shape, nipples, skin consistency, vascular patterns, cyclical alterations, occurrence of tenderness, cysts, masses, dimpling
4. appearance of a lesion—when, changes since then, any trauma, characteristics
5. surgery, biopsy, mammography, trauma—type and sequelae
6. SBE (self-breast examination)—how often, timing in cycle, method, findings
7. axillary lymph nodes—enlargement, tenderness, pain, cyclical changes, any change in deodorant or shaving injury
8. drugs that may influence breasts—oral contraceptives, cyclical estrogen therapy, antihypertensives, psychotropics

In addition, a review of other systems may be warranted based on presenting symptoms, family and personal history, or elaboration based on findings during the physical examination. For those clients taking or wanting to obtain oral contraceptives, review of cardiovascular, hemopoietic, respiratory, endocrine, and gastrointestinal systems would be appropriate to rule out contraindications.

Sample Write-up for History and Systems Review (all under S of SOAP [Subjective, Objective, Assessment, Plan] Notes)

Personal and social history
Barbara Smith
Storrs Road
Storrs, Connecticut
DOB 12/15/50, Hartford, Connecticut

Single, lives with friend in five-room apartment. Has a master's degree in special education; currently full-time doctoral student in special education at university; part-time employment at state school for children with special needs. Covered by student health insurance plan. Jogs two miles per day; swims and ice skates regularly (two to three times a week) and bicycles four or more times a week, weather permitting. Parents both are third-generation English-Americans. No pertinent cultural beliefs, customs, prohibitions.

Informant
  Self; appears reliable.

Family history
  Father has hypercholesterolemia, hypertension, on medication for B/P. Mother had a hysterectomy for bleeding (fibroids?) several years ago. Grandmother (maternal) had breast cancer and is deceased. Other grandparents died of "old age," other cause unknown. Siblings, two male, two female, alive and well. No family history of diabetes, varicosities, phlebitis, clotting disorders, migraines, allergies, CVA, venereal disease, or renal disease. Pregnancy and menstrual histories were normal as far as client is aware.

Personal medical history
  Never hospitalized, no injuries, no surgery. Illnesses confined to colds, strep throat "once or twice" when young—treated with penicillin. No history of rheumatic fever. Last immunizations at beginning of college— polio, DT. Has annual physical exam; sees dentist every year. Chicken pox, measles, mumps, and rubella as a child, no sequelae or complications. Denies any allergies.

Drug history
  Takes two to four Tylenol per month for headaches or cramps. No other OTC drugs or prescription meds. Takes 100 mg vitamin C per day. Does not smoke. One to two drinks per month (glass of wine, grasshopper at a party). Denies use of recreational drugs.

Diet history
  Weight since age 18 fluctuates between 120 and 124; height 5′ 5″. Sample day:

  Breakfast: 6 oz frozen orange juice, one egg, tea, whole wheat toast plain or ½ cup natural cereal with whole milk (approximately ½ cup)
  Lunch: one carton commercial yogurt or ½ cup homemade yogurt with fresh, dry, or frozen fruit; 1 oz cheese (Swiss, cheddar); one piece of fresh fruit (apple, pear, peach); tea with milk or 4–6 oz whole milk

Supper: one serving (½–1 cup) green or yellow fresh vegetable; 1–2 oz cheese, one or two eggs, or 4 oz fish, chicken, or meat; fresh fruit, cottage cheese, lettuce salad, creamy or oil and vinegar dressing; milk or tea or both

Snacks: fresh fruit, peanuts (not processed), ice cream, raisins, cookies, fruit juice, popcorn

Note: minimal use of salt, sugar, processed foods

Current complaint

"I think I have a vaginal infection—maybe yeast; I have had itching and burning for the past three days and increased discharge. I have never had this before, but have friends who have."

Systems review

Onset of menses age 11, cycles q. 28–35 days, some dysmenorrhea relieved by Tylenol, small clots, flow heavy for one day (four to six super tampons), duration three to four days. Some fluid retention and feeling "crabby"; notices mittelschmerz some months, urinary frequency at time of ovulation. LMP 2/17; no midcycle spotting, no pregnancies or abortions; no DES exposure; denies VD, any previous vaginal infections. Last Pap (1978) was negative. Contraception: on OC four years, some fluid retention, feeling "bloated and crabby"; wants to switch to diaphragm. Sexually active four to five times a week; no dyspareunia, orgasmic, denies postcoital bleeding; denies any urinary tract symptoms (frequency, burning, urgency, blood in urine).

Uses deodorant tampons, denies douching, denies use of deodorant sprays. Wears nylon underwear, often to bed. Measures laundry soap. Uses nonperfumed bath soap, no powder, no bubble bath. Often uses perfumed toilet paper.

Symptoms

Vaginal discharge increasing over past two to four days, vulva and vagina itchy, no odor to discharge. Denies any pain, masses, or lesions noted on genitals.

Breasts and lymphatics

Breast development at about age 12, no problems. Denies lumps, cysts, dimpling, changes in nipples, discharge, changes in pigmentation or areolae, trauma, surgery, biopsy, or mammography. Tenderness and slight enlargement noted before menses. Does SBE "once in a while," no special time of cycle. Denies enlargement, tenderness, or changes in axillary lymph nodes.

SELF-CHECK

1. List the components of a history and systems review for a gynecologic examination.
2. Do a write-up of an interview you conduct.

References

1. Bernstein L, Bernstein RS, Dana RH: *Interviewing: A Guide for Health Professionals*, ed 2. New York, Appleton-Century-Crofts, 1974, pp 33–37.
2. Daniel WA, Brown RT, Garrison CL: Adolescence: the clinical encounter and common health problems, in Mercer RT: *Perspectives on Adolescent Health Care.* Philadelphia, Lippincott, 1979, pp 147–171.
3. Trandel-Korenchuk DM, Trandel-Korenchuk KM: Minor consent in birth control and abortion, part 2. *Nurse Practitioner* 5: 48; 50; 54, 1980.
4. Trandel-Korenchuk DM, Trandel-Korenchuk KM: Minor consent in birth control and abortion, part 1. *Nurse Practitioner* 5: 47; 50–51; 54, 1980.
5. Futrell M, Brovender S, McKinnon-Mullett E, et al: *Primary Health Care of the Older Adult.* North Scituate, Mass, Duxbury Press, 1980, p 88.
6. Affonso DD: Framework for cultural assessment, in Clark AL, Affonso DD with Harris TR: *Childbearing: A Nursing Perspective.* ed. 2. Philadelphia: Davis, 1979, pp 117–118.
7. Branch MF, Paxton PP: *Providing Safe Nursing Care for Ethnic People of Color.* New York, Appleton-Century-Crofts, 1976, p 157.

For Futher Reading

Bates B: *A Guide to Physical Assessment*, ed 2. Philadelphia, Lippincott, 1979.

Berger K, Fields W: *Pocket Guide to Health Assessment.* Reston, Va, Reston Publishing, 1980.

Clark AL: *Culture Childbearing Health Professional.* Philadelphia, Davis, 1978.

Gillies DA, Alyn IB: *Patient Assessment and Management by the Nurse Practitioner.* Philadelphia, Saunders, 1976.

Green TH Jr: *Gynecology—Essentials of Clinical Practice*, ed 3. Boston, Little, Brown, 1977.

Prior JA, Silberstein JS: *Physical Diagnosis*, ed 5. St. Louis, CV Mosby, 1977.

Sherman JL Jr, Fields SK: *Guide to Patient Evaluation.* Flushing, NY, Medical Examination Publishing, 1974.

Spector R, *Cultural Diversity in Health and Illness.* New York, Appleton-Century-Crofts, 1979.

Review of Anatomy and Physiology

At the end of Chapter 2, you will be able to:

1. name and describe the function and processes of the structures of the female reproductive system
2. name and describe the functions and processes of the structures of the breast
3. describe the dynamics of the menstrual cycle, including hormones involved and their effects on the vagina, uterus, and ovaries

Pelvic Anatomy

The structures of the female reproductive system may be classified as internal and external.

External organs of reproduction

The external genitalia are collectively called the vulva and include the structures shown in Figure 2.1. The *mons pubis* is the fat pad that covers the symphysis. After puberty, pubic hair covers this area in a very definite pattern, which differs from that of the male. The hair grows in the shape of a triangle straight across the top of the pubic bone, tapering toward the groin and extending downward. It is not considered abnormal, however, for a woman to have a line of hair extending from the mons to the umbilicus.

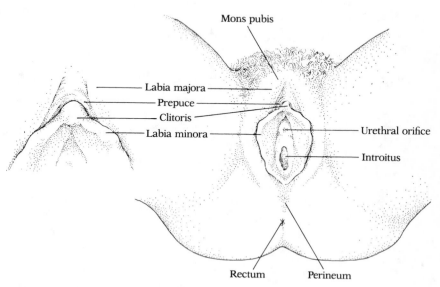

Figure 2.1   Vulva; Detail of Clitoris

13

The *labia majora* are outer folds of skin covering fat pads. They contain hair follicles on their outer surfaces and have highly pigmented inner surfaces. The *labia minora* are thinner folds of skin that contain many sebaceous glands. The anterior portions join to form the *prepuce* or hood of the clitoris. The two sets of labia are also called the inner and outer lips. The *clitoris* is a highly sensitive organ composed of erectile tissue.

The urinary opening, *urethral orifice* or *meatus*, is located between the clitoris and the introitus. In some women it appears as a small elevation of dimpled tissue. Paraurethral glands (skene's ducts) surround the urethra.

The *introitus* is the vaginal opening. The hymen is a fold of mucous membrane that normally covers (to varying degree) the opening of the vagina in a virgin. Hymenal skin tags may be seen around the vaginal introitus. Some hymen variations are shown in Figure 2.2. Bartholin's glands, located on either side of the introitus, help lubricate the vagina during sexual intercourse.

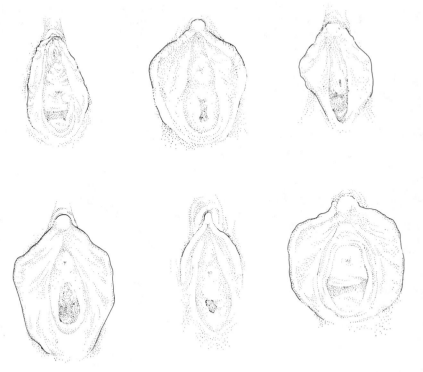

Figure 2.2   Hymen Variations

The *perineum* is the entire external pelvic floor from the mons to the coccyx. However, it is common to refer to the space between the posterior end of the introitus and the rectum as the perineum. The external genitalia may not be fully developed in an adolescent woman and may be atrophied in a woman who is postmenopausal.

Internal organs of reproduction

The internal female organs are show in Figures 2.3 and 2.4. They are the vagina, cervix, uterus, fallopian tubes, and ovaries.

The *vagina* is a musculomembranous tube-like organ situated between the uterus and external genitalia. A highly dilatable organ, it is ordinarily a potential space rather than an open cylinder or "hole." It is about seven to nine centimeters long with the anterior surface a bit shorter than the posterior. The vagina is posterior to the bladder and urethra and anterior to the rectum and anus. The cervix protrudes into the vagina forming four spaces: the anterior fornix, posterior fornix, and two lateral fornices.

The vaginal wall is composed of three layers: fascial, muscular, and mucous membrane. The innermost or mucous layer of squamous epithelium is arranged in folds or rugae, which tend to thin out or even disappear in the parous woman. The vagina contains few glands; how-

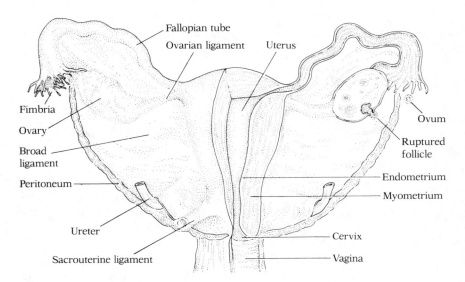

Figure 2.3   Internal Organs of Reproduction

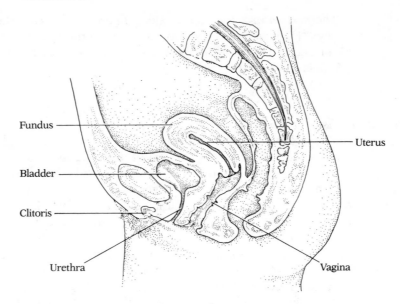

Fundus

Bladder

Clitoris

Urethra

Uterus

Vagina

Figure 2.4   Female Pelvic Organs—Side View

ever, secretions come from the mucous-producing cells, the cervix, and the bacteria normally present in the vagina.

The pH of the vagina is normally acidic (pH of four to six). This acid environment is protective in that it discourages growth of pathogenic organisms. The ability to maintain an acid pH is thought to be due to the activity of the lactobacilli on the glycogen contained in the cells of the mucous layer, which in turn acidifies the cervical mucus. The vaginal environment becomes slightly more alkaline just before and during menstruation. Because vaginal cells change in response to hormonal stimulation, they may be tested to determine hormonal activity and balance.

During copulation, this organ holds the penis and accepts sperm. Menstrual fluid and the fetus also pass through the vagina to the outside of the body.

The *cervix* is the neck of the uterus, of which the lower portion protrudes into the vagina and may be visualized during a pelvic exam. Its opening, the cervical canal or os, connects the uterus and vagina. On the uterine side, the opening is called the internal os while on the vaginal side it is called the external os.

Two types of epithelial tissue are found on the cervix. These are squamous epithelium, which covers the vagina and ectocervix, and columnar epithelium, which covers the endocervical canal surfaces. They meet near the external os at a point called the squamocolumnar junctions. The columnar epithelium may change into squamous epithelium forming a "transformation zone." Squamous metaplasia, as this transformation process is called, occurs primarily at three distinct developmental stages of a female's life. They are during fetal life, adolescence, and first pregnancy. Sometimes the process results in the formation of atypical cells rather than in normal squamous epithelium. Clinically this process results in the appearance of an ectropion (formerly termed an erosion).

The *uterus* is a hollow, muscular, pear-shaped organ, located in the pelvis, lying at right angles to the vagina, between the rectum posteriorly and the bladder anteriorly. It is a target organ responding to the secretions of the pituitary and ovaries. The portion of the uterus that lies above the insertion of the fallopian tubes is called the fundus. The thick walls of the uterus are comprised of three layers: the outer or serous layer, which is derived from the peritoneum; the middle muscular layer or myometrium, through which many blood vessels are intertwined; and the inner layer or endometrium, which is composed of epithelium, blood vessels, and glands. The endometrium, which is continuous with the mucous membrane of the vagina and fallopian tubes, is dynamic, responding to ovarian hormonal influences.

The uterus is not in a fixed position; rather it is suspended by ligaments, which are fibrous cords covered with peritoneum. The broad ligaments provide support for the ovaries and tubes in addition to the uterus. They also contain blood vessels, ovarian ligaments, nerves, and lymphatics. The other ligaments are the two round, two cardinal, and two uterosacral—one anterior and one posterior. The posterior ligament forms a pouch (cul-de-sac of Douglas) between the anterior surface of the rectum and the posterior surface of the uterus.

The uterus is endowed with an abundant blood supply, which reaches it via the internal iliac, inferior vena cava, and left renal veins.

The uterus functions to protect and nourish the growing fetus during pregnancy.

The *fallopian* or *uterine* tubes extend laterally from each side of the uterus. About eleven centimeters long and six millimeters in diameter, they are held in place by a portion of the broad ligament called the *mesosalpinx*. The distal end of each tube is funnel-shaped and fimbriated; these fimbriae help propel the egg released from the ovary into the tube, where fertilization may occur. The egg is then held in the tube for a few days before continuing its journey to the uterus. The ovum is moved by peristaltic action of the muscular layer of the tube and by the movement of the ciliated inner layer. The outer layer is serous.

The *ovaries* are almond-shaped organs about three centimeters in length, located on either side of the pelvis and lateral to the uterus. A fold of peritoneum, the mesovarian, suspends the ovary from the broad ligament. The ovarian ligament anchors it to the uterus. It is also attached to one of the fimbria of the fallopian tube.

The ovary has two parts: the inner part or medulla and the outer portion or cortex. The appearance of the outer surface of the ovary varies considerably with a women's maturity. Connective tissue, blood vessels, nerves, and lymphatic tissue are all found in the medulla. The cortex, covered by germinal epithelium, contains thousands of minute follicles. Each follicle contains a germ cell or oocyst. Every month an oocyte matures within a blister that forms on the surface of the ovary (see section on menstruation).

The ovaries are the essential organs of reproduction. They develop the ova and secrete estrogens and progesterones.

Nerve supply

The pelvic organs are innervated by both the autonomic and spinal nerve pathways. The branches of sacral nerves two, three, and four form the pudendal nerve, which supplies the external genitalia. The hyogastric and pelvic plexuses of the autonomic nervous system also supply the pelvis.

Blood supply

The arteries and veins supplying blood to the genital organs are illustrated in Figure 2.5.

Muscles

The complexity of muscles comprising the pelvic floor is illustrated in Figures 2.6 and 2.7.

Breasts

Female breasts, the most obvious sign of a women's physical and sexual maturity, enlarge during puberty under the influence of estrogen and progesterone. The breasts or mammary glands are considered accessory organs of reproduction because of their ability to manufacture milk for the nourishment of infants. The breasts are also highly erogenous; many women experience sensual pleasure during breast feeding and fondling the breasts is common during foreplay and masturbation. Breasts are also important to the self-image of most women. Although breast size

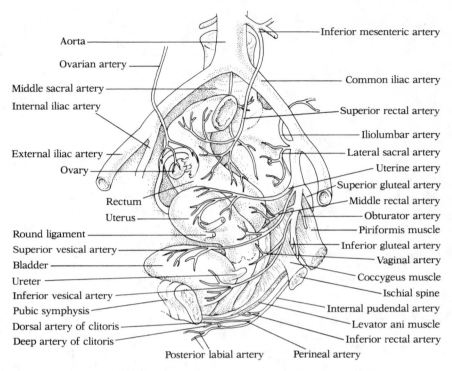

Aorta

Ovarian artery

Middle sacral artery

Internal iliac artery

External iliac artery

Ovary

Rectum

Uterus

Round ligament

Superior vesical artery

Bladder

Ureter

Inferior vesical artery

Pubic symphysis

Dorsal artery of clitoris

Deep artery of clitoris

Posterior labial artery

Inferior mesenteric artery

Common iliac artery

Superior rectal artery

Iliolumbar artery

Lateral sacral artery

Uterine artery

Superior gluteal artery

Middle rectal artery

Obturator artery

Piriformis muscle

Inferior gluteal artery

Vaginal artery

Coccygeus muscle

Ischial spine

Internal pudendal artery

Levator ani muscle

Inferior rectal artery

Perineal artery

Figure 2.5   Pelvic Blood Supply

varies a great deal from woman to woman, the size is not indicative of the ability to produce milk.

A young woman's breasts are relatively firm, with the nipple located on the same plane as the midpoint between elbow and shoulder. Breast development is a first sign of puberty. As aging occurs, the breasts become softer and the breast mass lowers. Fat decreases and fibrous tissue replaces glandular tissue.[1] Breast size increases slightly during the time just before menstruation each month because of hormonal influences. Breast size usually increases drastically during pregnancy and lactation.

Essentially, the breast is composed of glandular tissue, adipose or fat tissue, and connecting tissue. It extends from the second to the sixth rib and laterally from the sternum to the axilla. The glandular tissue is surrounded by fibrous tissue that, along with ligaments and underlying muscles, supports the breast. The muscles that lie beneath the breast are about two thirds of the pectoralis major and about one third of the serratus anterior. See Figure 2.8 for lymph nodes surrounding the breasts. The nipple of erectile tissue is located at the center of the breast and

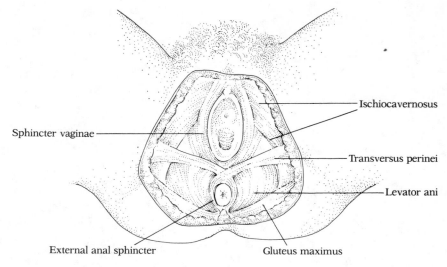

Sphincter vaginae

Ischiocavernosus

Transversus perinei

Levator ani

External anal sphincter

Gluteus maximus

Figure 2.6   Muscles of the Vulva and Pelvic Floor

contains 12 to 20 tiny openings, each of which leads to a lactiferous duct that arises from a glandular tissue lobe. The pigmented skin of the nipple, extending to the surface of the breast for a few centimeters surrounding the nipple, is called the areola. It contains many large sebaceous glands that lubricate the nipple helping to keep it supple during lactation.

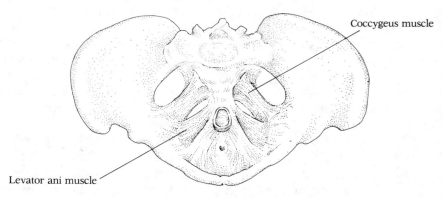

Coccygeus muscle

Levator ani muscle

Figure 2.7   Levatores Ani and Coccygei Muscles

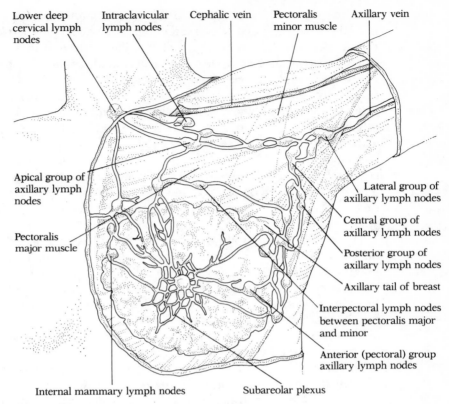

Figure 2.8   Lymphatic Drainage of the Breast

Menstruation

The ultimate purpose of the menstrual cycle is to enable childbearing. The process of menstruation begins during puberty and ends during the menopause. This section will examine four interwoven aspects of the menstrual cycle: hormonal, ovarian, uterine, and vaginal. Interrelated changes occur in the hormones and organs of reproduction. The menstrual cycle may vary between 20 and 45 days, but the 28-day cycle will be used for discussion purposes.

The hypothalamus secretes gonadotropin-releasing hormone (GRH), which causes the pituitary gland to release the gonadotropic luteinizing hormone (LH) and the follicle-stimulating hormone (FSH). Other hormones involved in the process are estrogen and progesterone. Stimulation, response, and feedback mechanisms cause changes in the reproductive organs, the pituitary gland, and the hypothalamus.

During the first part of the cycle, the hypothalamus increases secretion of GRH, which stimulates the secretion of FSH, which in turn stimulates the development of an ovarian follicle (one ovum and its surrounding cells). The ovarian follicle begins to grow rapidly at about the sixth day of the cycle and fills with fluid. This large blister-like projection off the surface of the ovary is called the graafian follicle. During its rapid growth, the follicle secretes increasingly greater amounts of estrogen, which inhibits the pituitary gland from secreting FSH. FSH, in turn, stops the ovaries from secreting estrogen. At about day 12 or 13, the pituitary releases LH, which causes the mature follicle to rupture. The egg is released into the abdominal cavity where it is caught by the fimbriated ends of the fallopian tube and is conveyed through the tube to the uterus. The egg, after bursting forth from the graafian follicle, has a life span of about 24 hours.

The portion of the follicle still in the ovary fills with blood, is sealed off, and becomes the corpus hemorrhagicum and then the corpus luteum, which consists of secretory cells. These cells secrete estrogen and progesterone. The least estrogenic and predominant estrogen during pregnancy is estriol. If fertilization of the ovum does not occur, the corpus luteum grows for two more weeks and then disintegrates and is absorbed. The only indication of its past existence is a scar it leaves on the ovary, called the corpus albicans.

The uterine lining is also in a dynamic state during this ovarian-pituitary cycle. The endometrium or uterine lining, without the support of estrogen and progesterone, begins to shed and passes to the outside of the body via the vagina to become the menstrual flow. The menstrual fluid (about 100 ml) consists of mucin, blood, and epithelial cells. This lasts from day one to about day five of the menstrual cycle.

The *proliferative* phase of the cycle lasts from day five to day 14. This phase occurs during the development of the rapidly growing follicle, which is secreting estrogen. The blood supply of the uterus is increased as is the deposition of glycogen, lipids, water, and electrolytes, causing the uterine lining to thicken.

Following ovulation the *secretory* phase occurs with the production and secretion of progesterone by cells of the corpus luteum. The lining of the uterus continues to prepare for the fertilized ovum and increases to about a five-millimeter thickness by day 24. During this time the corpus luteum is disintegrating, and the levels of estrogen and progesterone are dropping. A shrinking in the uterine lining occurs because of a loss of fluid in the surface layers. The blood supply decreases and causes some necrotic areas in the endometrium. Sloughing occurs into the uterine cavity by day 28 and a new cycle is imminent, heralded by the *menstrual* phase.

Cyclical changes also occur in the vagina. During the estrogen-dominated first half of the menstrual cycle, the pH of the vagina is about 4.5 and dried mucus viewed under a microscope shows a ferning pattern. During the second half of the cycle, the mucus secretions thicken, the environment tends to be more alkaline, and the mucus sample does not show the fern-like quality. One can then assume that ovulation has occurred.

Changes during menarche

During puberty, a girl's body undergoes many changes that signal the menarche or onset of menstruation. The earliest signs are usually the budding of breasts and the appearance of pubic hair. It is not unusual for these to occur as young as age 9. The reproductive organs, both internal and external, grow and change gradually until they resemble those of a mature woman in both size and shape. Axillary hair then appears, followed by menarche. The age of menarche varies a great deal: the average is 13 or 14 but it may occur as late as 17. The menstrual cycles may occur at uneven intervals for a few years or more with the first few anovulatory.

Evidence suggests that an increasing amount of gonadotropin-releasing factor (GRF) initiates puberty. This hormone is a product of the nuclei of the hypothalamus.[2] The predominant estrogen in pubescent women is estradiol. The stimulation of the body by estrogen is reflected in the distribution of fat and by epiphyseal closures, completing bone growth. Maximum height is achieved by about the 18th year. The five to one ratio of muscle to fat before puberty changes to about three to one after puberty.

Changes during the climacteric

The climacteric is the period of time, usually about 15 years, in which the estrogen produced by the ovaries decreases. The predominant estrogen after menopause is estrone. Estrone can be derived from peripheral conversion of androstenedione. Menopause, the cessation of menses, also may occur gradually. A woman should consider that she is still fertile until she has not menstruated for one year.

The decreasing estrogen production may cause some common physical manifestations. They may appear as vasomotor irregularities, for example, the hot flush (hot flash). This is a blushing sensation that usually begins at the waist and moves progressively upward to the head. Profuse perspiration may occur at the completion of the flush. Other symptoms are tingling of the hands and feet, dizziness, headaches, and palpitations. The bones may begin to lose calcium, a condition known as osteoporosis.

The walls of the vagina may become thin and dry. Lubrication in the vagina decreases. The amount of fat in the mons decreases with aging, as does the amount, color, and texture of pubic hair. Labia often atrophy.[3]

Sexual dysfunction may occur, not necessarily as a direct result of the menopause but rather of society's view of menopause and, ultimately, the woman's view of herself. Anatomic and physiologic changes, however, may alter sexual response. An understanding of changes related to menopause and the aging process will enable the woman to continue to enjoy her sexuality.

SELF-CHECK

Becky's mother brought her to see the nurse because she was concerned about her daughter's development. Becky is 14 years old and even though her breasts have begun to develop she still has not begun to menstruate. Becky's mother reached menarche at age 12.

1. What would your approach be?
2. What patterns of change occur in the female body at puberty?
3. What hormones are involved in these changes?
4. Diagram and label the female reproductive organs. For each organ, describe anatomy and function. Discuss the blood, nerve, and muscle supplies of the female pelvis.

When Maria Cortez visited the nurse practitioner, she stated that for about six months her periods had been very irregular and she had not menstruated for two months. Maria is 48 years old and has two concerns. First, could she be pregnant? Second, if she is not pregnant could she discontinue the use of contraceptives, assuming that she has probably been through menopause?

1. How would you answer Maria's questions?
2. What other things would you discuss with Maria?

References

1. McKenzie CA: Sexuality and the menopausal woman. *Issues in Health Care of Women* 1: 39, 1978.

2. Tichy AM, Malasanos LJ: The physiological role of hormones in puberty. *The American Journal of Maternal Child Nursing* 1: 384, 1976.
3. Futrell M, Brovender S, McKinnon-Mullett E, et al: *Primary Health Care of the Older Adult.* North Scituate, Mass, Duxbury Press, 1980, p 197.

For Further Reading

Bates B: *A Guide to Physical Assessment,* ed 2. Philadelphia, Lippincott, 1979.
Gray H: *Anatomy, Descriptive and Surgical,* 1901 ed. Philadelphia, Running Press, 1974.
Novak ER, Jones GS, Jones HW: *Gynecology,* ed 9. Baltimore, Williams & Wilkins, 1975.

Techniques of Examination

At the end of Chapter 3, you will be able to delineate, assess, and evaluate the following:

1. equipment needed for the gynecologic examination
2. rationale for selection of the type of speculum
3. type of lubricant used and when used
4. proper media for smears and/or cultures for gonorrhea, Trichomonas, Candida, herpes, and other commonly found organisms and techniques for obtaining and handling specimens
5. equipment necessary to do a Pap smear and the process for care of the specimen once obtained

Prior to examination of a client, it is helpful to assemble the equipment needed for that examination. It is preferable to have a setting that affords privacy and is equipped with a gynecologic exam table, a stool for the examiner, and a light that can be adjusted to visualize the perineum, vagina, and cervix.

The supplies described in this section are those specific to the gynecologic examination. In addition, of course, a stethoscope, ophthalmoscope, otoscope, tongue depressor, tuning fork, percussion hammer, eye chart, skin pencil, blood pressure cuff, ruler, and tape measure may be needed if a complete physical examination is to be performed as part of the assessment process.

Speculums

There are two main types of vaginal speculums utilized for a gynecologic examination in an ambulatory setting, metal and plastic. Metal speculums can be sterilized and reused while plastic speculums are designed for single use and disposal (see Figure 3.1). Each of the major types of speculums, the Pederson and the Graves, comes in three sizes. The Pederson speculum comes in large (2.5 x 12 cm), medium or regular (2.2 x 10 cm), and small (1.3 x 7.5 cm). The blades are narrower than those of

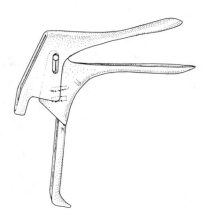

Figure 3.1 Disposable Speculum

the Graves and do not flare at the ends (see Figures 3.2 and 3.3). The Graves speculum comes in small (infant) size (1.9 x 7.5 cm), medium or regular (3.5 x 10 cm), and large (3.5 x 12 cm).

A speculum consists of two parts, the blades and the handle. The blades are inserted in the vagina and then gently opened or separated by use of the lever to spread the vaginal walls and allow for visualization of the walls, fornices, and cervix. The handle remains on the outside, allowing the examiner to manipulate the speculum easily. The thumb screw on the handle at the base of the blades allows the blades to be spread widely to increase visibility, and the thumb screw on the lever locks the blades open to free both hands of the examiner for doing the Pap smear and other procedures.

The speculum may be warmed prior to use by running it under warm water or by having a heating pad or other heat-producing device such as a light in the drawer or wherever the speculums are kept.

Selection of the type and size of speculum to be used is based on an assessment of the following: physical and sexual maturity of client, use of tampons and length of time used, status of the hymen, duration of sexual activity (months, years), pregnancy history, and visual inspection of the introitus and perineum. If the woman's hymen appears to be intact or partially intact and if she has never been examined before, a medium Pederson might be chosen. If the woman has been sexually active for some time, has used tampons for years, and/or has had a pregnancy, a medium Graves or a large Pederson might be the choice. For a woman whose introitus appears large and who has been sexually active and had several pregnancies, a large Graves speculum might be chosen.

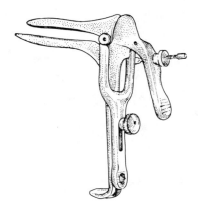

Figure 3.2   Pederson Speculum

It should be noted that there is slightly less size variation with disposable speculums, most of which resemble a modified Graves/Pederson. There are three sizes available: small, medium, and large. These speculums have sliding notched lever and blade width adjustments rather than thumb screws. The examiner should be particularly attentive to insertion and removal since the sliding lock arrangement makes it easy to catch pubic hair or labial skin folds.

Gloves

Sterilized surgical gloves may be used during the exam. More commonly, disposable prepowdered gloves of clear or colored plastic are used; they are designed to fit either hand and available in sizes small to extra large in dispenser boxes or wrapped singly. Because the vagina is a clean and not a sterile orifice, gloves used are generally clean, following principles of medical asepsis. Should maintenance of a sterile field be desirable, such as during insertion of an intrauterine device, a pair of sterile surgical gloves is preferable. Sterile gloves are also used in some venereal disease clinics and when there is any chance of direct contamination of the uterus or its contents.

Lubricant

The type of lubricant utilized is a clear, colorless, water-soluble gel that is easily removed from instruments, skin, and clothing. It should never be used when obtaining a Pap smear, cultures, or smears for organisms as it

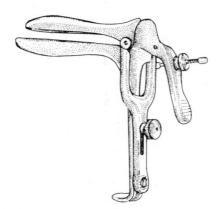

Figure 3.3   Graves Speculum

will interfere with laboratory results. Water or saline may be used to warm and lubricate the speculum for insertion when a Pap smear or other smear or culture is to be done. The gel lubricant may then be used for the bimanual and rectal examinations. This same lubricant may be recommended to clients for use during intercourse when natural lubrication is insufficient for comfortable penetration and thrusting.

Pap Smear Equipment

Equipment necessary to perform a Papanicolaou (Pap) smear may include a special Pap stick of wood or plastic, slide for the specimen, container for the slide, fixative agent, swab for endocervical specimen, and possibly glass pipette and rubber suction bulb for obtaining a specimen of the vaginal pool (see Figure 3.4). If the woman is menstruating or bleeding for any reason, the Pap smear should be deferred since it will be distorted by the presence of blood. The woman should also not have douched for 24 hours or used contraceptive jelly, cream, or foam for 24 to 48 hours. When the specimen is obtained from the cervical os, surface of the cervix, and vaginal pool, it is spread on the glass slide and then either immersed in the ether and alcohol fixative or sprayed with it and placed in a protective cardboard slide container or envelope. Some laboratories use hair spray as a fixative. Slides usually have a frosted end upon which the client's name and any other identifying data may be

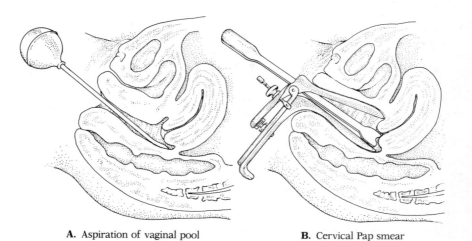

A. Aspiration of vaginal pool   B. Cervical Pap smear

Figure 3.4   Pap Smear Technique

written in pencil. Some glass slides are divided into three sections, one each for endocervical, cervical, and vaginal specimens.

A Schiller's test may be routinely performed in some settings. This test involves use of Schiller's solution, composed of 1 part iodine, 2 parts potassium iodide, and 300 parts water. This solution is either poured into the vagina or painted on the cervix. Normal cells will take up the dye evenly; abnormal cells will not, causing light-colored areas to appear.[1(pp 17–18, 28–29)]

The maturation index, important to endocrine evaluation, may also be obtained from vaginal epithelial cell samples. The maturation index is descriptive of the percentage of parabasal, intermediate, and superficial cells in a smear. Previously this was called the cornification index and the cell types parabasal, cornified, and precornified. A maturation index indicating marked estrogen effect might look like this:

$$0 \quad / \quad 10 \quad / \quad 90$$
$$\text{parabasal} \quad \text{intermediate} \quad \text{superficial}$$

Over 30% of superficial cells indicates marked estrogen effect. If more than 50% parabasal cells are present, estrogen effect is low. It should be noted that infection or inflammation may distort the index.[1(pp21–22)]

Media for Smears, Samples, and Cultures

The medium necessary for smears and cultures is often specific to the organism one suspects. In screening for Trichomonas and Candida albicans, both a dry smear on a slide or a wet smear in saline may be done. The wet smear may be sent to the lab either in a sterile culture tube with saline added or on a slide with a cover slip. Nickerson's medium, which comes in a small tube, can also be used to identify Candida when diagnosis is in doubt from a wet smear.[1(pp24–25)] Yeast buds can be identified using a 10 to 20% solution of KOH (potassium hydroxide). This solution dissolves cellular debris and the yeast buds will remain (see Figure 3.5).[2(p206)]

In men, gonorrhea can be identified with a smear. For women, this is not an accurate method. A culture should be grown on the Thayer-Martin medium, which is enriched blood or chocolate agar. This culture is taken with a sterile swab, painted on the medium, and then a tablet of carbon dioxide is added and the specimen sealed in a plastic bag.[2(pp205–206)] A candle jar can be used when Thayer-Martin medium with carbon dioxide tablets is not available.

During history taking, modes of exposure should be explored. If oral sex is practiced, it is important to culture the nasopharynx, the anus, and

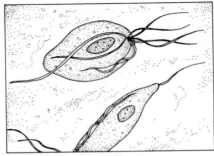

A. Trichomonas vaginalis   **B.** Candida hyphac and yeast buds

Figure 3.5   Vaginal Smears

the cervix. The anal area can be contaminated by vaginal secretions and semen, as well as by direct contact during intercourse. Specimens are usually labeled as to site and time obtained to ensure proper handling and incubation and to aid in diagnosis and interventions.

Herpes virus is detectable by doing a herpes virus type 2 antibody titer when active lesions are present and then obtaining a convalescent titer ten days later. These require blood samples, usually drawn by a lab technician, although you may be the person to do so. A Pap smear of the lesion will show the characteristic multinucleation. A culture may be done and placed on Eagle's medium, specific for herpes virus.

The Frei test, an antigen skin test, specific to the virus, is used to rule out lymphogranuloma venereum.

A gram stain smear can be done to diagnose chanchroid, which is caused by a gram negative coccus bacillus. Giemsa stain and Wright's stain are used for granuloma inguinala and molluscum contagiosum. A wet smear with sodium chloride can be used for diagnosis of hemophilus vaginalis. Specimens for any of these may be placed on slides with cover slips and protected for transport to the lab, or sterile culture tubes may be used.

When bacterial infections are suspected, sterile culture tubes containing swabs may be used to obtain and protect the specimens. Smears and stains may be read immediately for identification of organisms. Cultures generally take 24 to 72 hours or more to grow.

Chlamydia trachomatis, an intracellular parasite, requires special culture technique. A swab of the endocervical epithelium is taken and must be injected into culture medium immediately. In most cases, immediate injection is not possible, so a buffered holding medium of sucrose phosphase is used and the specimen is frozen at −7 C until injection can occur. Culturing the organism requires three to five days.

Having the proper media for cultures and equipment for smears ready, along with materials necessary for the physical aspects of the gynecologic health assessment will save you and your clients time and avoid repeat visits. A careful history will help you to ascertain which laboratory studies are appropriate and which data you need to collect. Knowledge of proper techniques for smears and cultures will prevent repetition of costly laboratory studies and aid in prompt diagnosis and intervention.

A fern test may also be done with a sample of mucus from the endo-cervix obtained with a dry glass pipette or a cotton-tipped applicator. After air drying for 10 to 20 minutes on a slide, the sample is examined under a microscope. A distinct ferning pattern will be present when adequate amounts of estrogen are present, thus before ovulation in the estrogen-dominated first half of the endometrial cycle. Progesterone obliterates this finding. This test is useful in determining whether or not ovulation has occurred, as well as in evaluation of quality of ovarian hormones (see Figure 3.6).[1(pp26–27)]

Although scrapings from primary and secondary lesions of syphilis may be examined for the spirochete under a dark-field microscope, it is usual and more reliable to screen for the disease using a venous blood specimen for serologic diagnosis.[2(p206)]

SELF-CHECK

Susan Smith comes in for a pelvic examination and Pap smear. She is 18 years old, has had intercourse only once, has used tampons for approximately one year, and has never been examined before. She also wants to be checked for venereal disease.

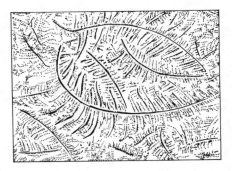

Figure 3.6 Characteristic Ferning of Vaginal Secretions at Mid-cycle

1. Which speculum would you choose on the basis of data given?
2. How will you evaluate your choice?
3. When will you use a lubricant and what type?
4. What equipment will you need for the examination?
5. What things do you need to do to screen for venereal disease?
6. What equipment would you assemble and which speculum would you select for the client in Chapter 1?

References

1. Green TH Jr: *Gynecology—Essentials of Clinical Practice,* ed 3. Boston, Little, Brown, 1977.
2. Widmann FK: *Goodale's Clinical Interpretation of Laboratory Tests,* ed 7. Philadelphia, Davis, 1973.

For Further Reading

Wallach, J: *Interpretation of diagnostic tests,* ed 3. Boston, Little, Brown, 1978.
Olson, BK: Patient comfort during pelvic examination: new foot supports vs metal stirrups. *Journal of Obstetric, Gynecologic and Neonatal Nursing* **10:** 104–107, 1981.

The Examination

At the end of Chapter 4, you will be able to:

1. describe and evaluate the steps of the gynecologic examination
2. evaluate rationale for observations and techniques included in this examination
3. analyze common aberrations of the external genitalia
4. describe the appearance of the cervix
5. list and define classes of Pap smears
6. synthesize findings of an examination in writing up SOAP notes

The gynecologic examination may be viewed as the most intimate and invasive component of a health assessment. Women have characterized the examination as embarrassing, completely terrifying, painful, and impersonal.[1] Cultural taboos and beliefs will affect the woman's view of the pelvic examination. She may be reluctant to have an examination before marriage or to be examined by a man. Most genital approaches are sexual so the gynecologic examination has overtones of intimacy and sexuality.

A setting that is formal and sterile does not easily promote relaxation and comfort. A cold examining table and speculum, impersonal disposable drape, and assuming the dorso-lithotomy position may make the woman feel both uncomfortable and vulnerable. Obviously many aspects of the physical environment can be altered to make the setting more comfortable and personal and less threatening. Soft-colored sheets for drapes, a warm room, warm speculum, covers on the stirrups, posters on the wall, raising the head of the table 30 to 60 degrees, and assurance of privacy will all help the woman to relax.

The attitude of the provider, however, is even more important in making the gynecologic examination a positive experience. Women today are seeking health care that is nonsexist, sensitive, and respectful. They want to be treated as intelligent human beings and to be given information that will help them take charge of their bodies and decision making.[2] Most of all, women indicate a strong preference for being cared for by women, especially for gynecologic care.[3]

The first pelvic examination is probably critical to the development of attitudes toward health care and gynecologic care in particular. The gynecologic examination may be a woman's first contact with the health-care delivery system without parental presence and support. Further, the examination by its very nature involves issues of sexuality, intimacy, body image, and identity.[1] Women indicate a strong need to know more about the methods and goals of the exam prior to its occurrence.[4] Encourage the woman to bring a friend for support if she wishes. Be sure to allow sufficient time for questions and discussion during the examination. As a provider of health care for women, your sensitivity and concern can make the experience as positive as possible.

36

Conducting the Examination

A private place to undress, a safe place to put clothes, and a soft, adequate drape will help the woman to feel more comfortable for the examination. Whereas a college-age woman may be unconcerned about a drape, a modest teenager may be very shy about her body.[5] The older woman, undergoing body changes associated with menopause and aging, may also be self-conscious about her body and need to have adequate time to undress and prepare for the examination. Simple, clear instructions will help to avoid embarrassment of not knowing what is expected. Prior to the examination, offer the woman a chance to empty her bladder. Tell her if you want a urine specimen and instruct her.

Gynecologic examination of a client begins with assisting her to a comfortable position with knees bent and with feet in stirrups or flat on the examining table. Factors such as age, size, culture, physical status, limitations in mobility, and symptoms will influence the amount of assistance she will require and modifications in position you may make. If possible, the woman's buttocks should be at the very edge of the table to facilitate insertion of the speculum. Her knees should be relaxed and dropped to the sides as far as is comfortable. This position helps to relax the vulva and perineum, maximize her comfort, and facilitate the examination. Drape the woman in a manner that is comfortable to her and convenient for you.

Explain each step of the examination as you proceed. Explanations of the procedures and reasons for them help the woman to relax and minimize her fear of the unknown, particularly if it is the first pelvic examination.

External Genitalia

After putting gloves on one or both hands, inspect the labia minora and major, carefully separating the two to check for lesions and signs of irritation. Retract the hood of the clitoris slightly to check for lesions, adhesions, and irritation. The labia should be palpated gently for nodules, irregularities, and lesions.

Using a good light, check the mons pubis for infestation of lice or other vermin, nits, lesions, sores, chancres, rash, and irritation. Palpate gently for nodules. A magnifying glass can be used to verify presence of nits or lice and a pubic hair may be inspected under the microscope.

Inspect the urethral orifice for purulent discharge, irritation, and fissures. Observe the hymenal ring and hymenal tags (remnants of hymen) for any fissures or lesions. Check and palpate the perineum for lesions and around the anal area for lesions, fissures, discharge, or hemorrhoids.

Gently press the area of Skene's (paraurethral) and Bartholin's glands to detect any swelling or tenderness. In postmenopausal women, the vagina may be atrophic or the walls very thin, and/or irritation around the urethra may be present necessitating very gentle insertion of the speculum.

Internal Examination

Prior to inserting the speculum, it may be helpful to instruct the woman in relaxation breathing, either long, slow, deep abdominal breathing or slow chest breathing. Both of these types of breathing, which are similar to yoga techniques, are used for prepared childbirth. Pressure on the cervix may trigger a vasovagal reaction, so observe the woman for pallor, perspiring, and other signs of syncope. Have ammonia ampules available in case she faints.

Inspection

The internal examination involves speculum inspection and bimanual palpation. If the speculum is warmed with water, test the temperature on the woman's inner thigh before inserting. The following is but one of a number of equally good techniques for insertion of the speculum. As a practitioner, in time you will develop a technique that is comfortable for you and your client. Gently insert the index finger of one hand into the introitus and press down gently on the pubococcygeal muscle. Then, withdrawing the index finger, spread the labia gently. Holding the closed blades of the speculum between the index and middle fingers of the other hand, insert the speculum so the blades are in a vertical position (see Figure 4.1). Never press anteriorally as the urethra is very sensitive. Once the speculum is inserted to the full extent of the blades (unless you meet resistance or cause pain), gently rotate so the blades are horizontal and the handle is pointing toward the floor. Carefully guide both insertion and rotation so that you do not pinch the labia or pull on pubic hairs.

Press the lever and open the blades slowly, maneuvering the speculum so that you can visualize the cervix (see Figure 4.2). If the uterus is retroverted, you may have to retract the speculum partway and reinsert it, angling more anteriorally. The reverse is true if the uterus is anteverted, as the cervix may be deep in the posterior fornix (see Figures 4.3, 4.4 and 4.5).

Once you have adjusted the speculum blades for visualization of the cervix, tighten the thumb screw on the lever. Adjust the light so you can inspect the cervix. It should appear bright pink or rosy, shiny, and

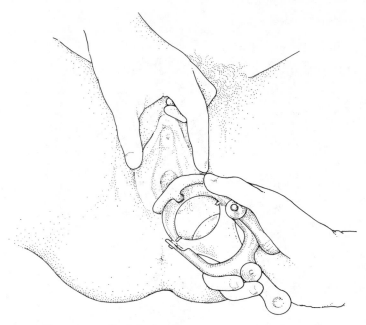

Figure 4.1   Insertion of Speculum

smooth. If the woman is nulliparous, the os will be circular or oval; if she is parous, it will be a slit (see Figures **4.6** and **4.7**). The os should be closed, although it will be slightly dilated during menses.

Offer the woman the opportunity to see her cervix, adjusting the light and using a hand-held mirror. Women report positive feelings toward the gynecologic examination when they are offered this experience.[6]

Pap smear

A Pap smear may be done using any one of a number of methods. A sterile cotton tipped swab can be used to obtain a specimen from the cervical os. The special wooden or plastic Pap stick is rotated over the surface of the cervix with the longer flange in the os, to scrape a sample of cells. The vaginal pool in the posterior fornix is sampled with a swab, the handle of the Pap stick, or a glass pipette and rubber bulb to aspirate the specimen. A single slide can be prepared; three separate slides, one from each area; or a three-part slide marked for each specimen: endo-cervical, cervical, and vaginal. It is important to use a single motion to put the specimen on the slide. A back-and-forth motion can destroy or distort cells. Check to see that a sufficient specimen is deposited on the

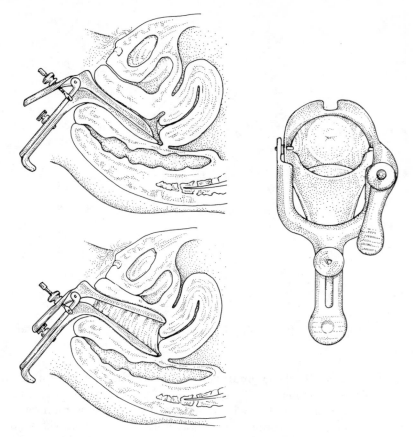

Figure 4.2   Opening Speculum and Visualizing Cervix

slide, spray or immerse the slide in fixative, and attach laboratory slips securely to the slide container.

Accuracy of Pap smears and avoidance of false negatives can be achieved through careful technique. Since the squamous-columnar junction is the site at which carcinoma is most likely to occur, identified by a margin of smooth pink squamous tissue meeting the darker pink rough columnar tissue, take a representative sample from this area.[7] A cotton-tipped applicator can be used to sample the endocervical canal or a cervical aspirator. The vaginal pool may be sampled, but should be only one of three samples, as it has a high false negative rate when used alone. Irrigation samples also are inadequate.[8]

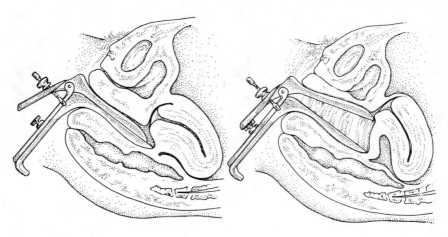

Figure 4.3   Retroverted Uterus

Immediate fixing of the slide is necessary so exposure to air will not distort cell quality. There are arguments for and against each kind of fixative. Sprays permeate poorly but are convenient, whereas bottles of 100% alcohol or formalin and carbo-wax liquid penetrate well, but are cumbersome.[9]

Once the Pap smear has been taken, along with any other smears or cultures you wish to obtain, loosen the thumb screw, and as you slowly close the blades, rotate the speculum to inspect the vagina. Note any lesions, discharge (color, character, odor), any irregularities, unusual color, and any signs of masses, irritation, or erythema. Remove the speculum gently with blades completely closed.

Bimanual

The bimanual examination allows you to palpate the vagina, ovaries (when possible), and uterus and to detect masses in the adnexa. Utilize a water-soluble jelly lubricant to make the examination as comfortable as possible and tell the woman that your fingers may feel cool or cold. With palm down, place the index and middle fingers of the internal examining hand in the introitus and then gently advance them into the vagina to the extent of their length. If you meet resistance or cause the client pain, readjust your hand. It may be necessary to use only one finger if the hymen is tight or the vaginal walls are very tense. Palpate the walls of the vagina and the fornices to detect any nodules or other lesions that may not have been visible or were obscured by the speculum.

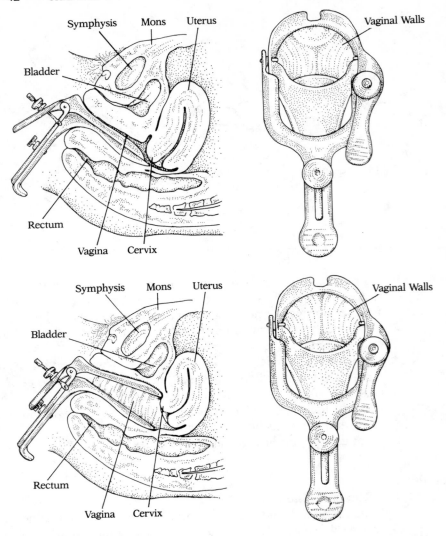

Figure 4.4   Anteverted Uterus

The external hand is used to palpate through the lower abdominal wall. Rotate your internal hand to a palm-up position and reach to the right adnexa while your external hand presses gently against the internal (see Figure 4.8). Attempt to palpate the right ovary and check for any masses. This is repeated on the left. In the midline, attempt to palpate the cervix and uterus with the internal hand and the corpus and fundus

with the external (see Figure 4.9). The position of the uterus will determine how much of the uterus you will feel. The uterus may be along an
axis with the vagina (midline position), tipped posteriorly toward the
sacrum (retroverted), anteverted toward the symphysis pubis, folded
into the cul-de-sac (retroflexed), or in an extreme anterior flexion (anteflexed) (see Figure 4.10). In addition, it may be dextro- or levorotated,
rotated to the right or the left, respectively. By palpating in the four fornices, different portions of the uterus can be felt, determined by its position.

Rarely, the fallopian tubes are palpable in a thin client. If they are
easily palpable, they may be enlarged by ectopic pregnancy or tumor.
The ovaries are almond-shaped and normally do not exceed four centimeters in length. They should feel relatively firm.

Finally, you should feel for bulges in the anterior wall of the vagina
(cystocele) and the posterior wall (rectocele) with the internal hand (see
Figure 4.10). After withdrawal of the hand to the introitus, spread your
fingers at the hymenal ring and have the woman bear down. Observe
for any bulging in the anterior or posterior vaginal wall.

For the woman who has had a hysterectomy, you will need to ascertain whether her cervix and/or ovaries are still present. If the cervix is
present, a Pap should be done annually and if not, a smear of vaginal
cells still may be done as a screening for vaginal carcinoma. A bimanual
examination should be done to detect any adnexal masses, and to palpate ovaries, if present, for enlargement or masses. A rectal examination
should be done to check for rectocele, cystocele, masses, and occult
blood.

Rectal

Leaving your index finger in the vagina, insert your middle finger gently in the anal orifice (see Figure 4.11). Pressure with the pad of your
finger against the sphincter will help insertion. Palpate the wall between
the rectum and vagina for any lesions, bulges, or fistulae. Rotate your
finger in the rectum 360 degrees to palpate for masses. Note the tone of
the sphincter muscle and ask the client to bear down to relax the muscle.
There is test material available to check for occult blood following the
rectal exam. It usually requires only that the examiner wipe the gloved
finger on the test material.

It is courteous to offer the woman tissues or a perineal wipe to remove
lubricant prior to getting dressed. Always allow the woman time to dress
before discussing findings, so she can sit comfortably and talk face to
face.

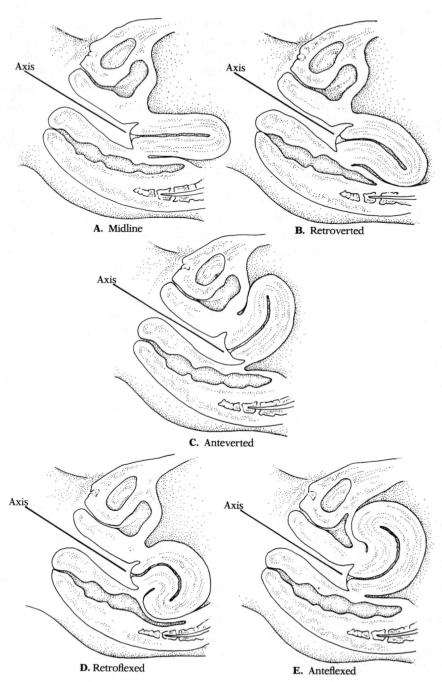

A. Midline

B. Retroverted

C. Anteverted

D. Retroflexed

E. Anteflexed

Figure 4.5 Positions of Uterus

44

Sample Write-up for History and Systems Review

Personal and social history

Marie Valdarez is a 57-year-old woman who lives with her husband, Salvatore, on the first floor of a three-family house in an older, well-kept neighborhood in the greater metropolitan area of Boston. They rent out the third-floor apartment, and their daughter and family live on the second floor. They have health insurance through Mr. Valdarez's employment. She gets no regular exercise other than walking a lot: "I don't drive so I walk to the markets to do my errands." Ms. Valdarez and her

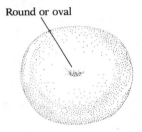

Round or oval

Figure 4.6   Nulliparous Cervix

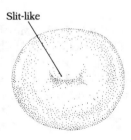

Slit-like

Figure 4.7   Parous Cervix

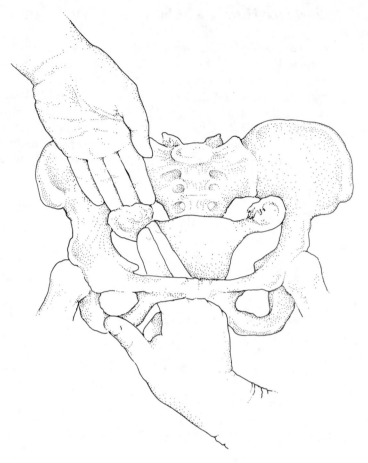

Figure 4.8   Bimanual Examination of Adnexa

husband came to the United States from Italy as small children and met in high school. They speak both Italian and English fluently. Ms. Valdarez says she does not like being examined and finds it embarrassing. She characterizes herself and her family as being Americans, "But we have our heritage and attend the Italian Catholic parish church and Italian social club."

Informant
    Self; appears reliable.

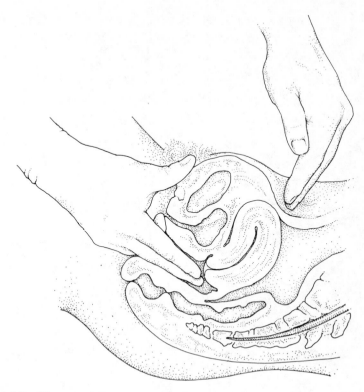

Figure 4.9   Bimanual Examination of Uterus

Family history

Ms. Valdarez's father and mother both died of CVAs in their 70s. Both had hypertension. Her sister died of breast cancer at 61 years of age. All five of her other siblings are alive and well. There is no family history of diabetes, varicosities, phlebitis, migraines, allergies, or venereal or renal disease.

Personal medical history

Hospitalized for the births of her children and in 1968 for a hysterectomy "for fibroid tumors." Illnesses: had usual childhood illnesses (chicken pox, measles, mumps, German measles, whooping cough). Vaccinated for smallpox as child; does not remember others—no recent immunizations. Some topical allergies.

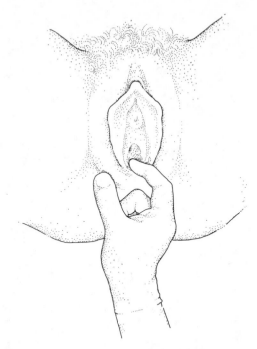

Figure 4.10   Palpation for Cystocele and Rectocele

Drug history

Uses several aspirin a month (maybe a dozen) for occasional arthritis, does not smoke, has wine (one glass four or five times a week), no other alcohol. Uses cathartics when needed (MOM or castor oil) once or twice a month. Uses antacid tablets for occasional heartburn and OTC medication to sleep (once a week maybe). Denies use of any other drugs.

Diet history

Weight 165, height 5′ 2″. Weight stable for past several years. Sample day:

Breakfast: coffee (two cups), toast (white bread)—two or three pieces, bran cereal (½ cup) with skim milk

Lunch: coffee (two cups), fresh fruit, vegetable (raw), sandwich (white bread) with bologna, salami, cheese, tomato, and lettuce

Supper: meat and potatoes or pasta and sauce; eggplant or other vegetables—squash, chard; fresh fruit, sometimes pastries; usually has bread (white), coffee, and small glass of wine

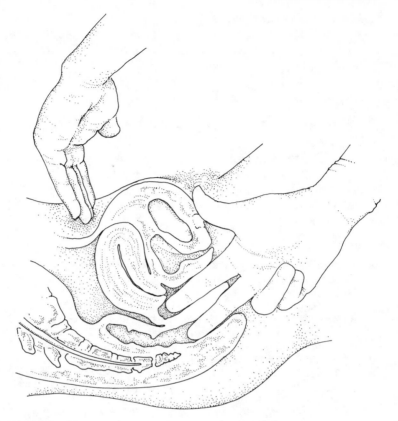

Figure 4.11   Bimanual Examination with Rectal Exam

Current complaint

Pain, itching, burning in vaginal area. "Don't feel like sex because it hurts." "Time for a check-up."

Systems review

Onset of menses age 12, cycles were regular "every month." Three pregnancies, last one twins. No complications except twins were two weeks early. Menstruated until hysterectomy—now has "hot flashes" occasionally but no other symptoms. Last Pap smear was "a couple of years ago and was okay." Sexually active once a month or so. Some problems—"seems to hurt and I seem dry"; also some itching "down there" and some burning "when urine comes out." Denies blood in urine, any bladder pain, or frequency. Wears underwear to bed, uses bubble bath sometimes and "lots" of baby powder.

Breasts and lymphatics

Bottle fed children. Denies any tenderness, cysts, bumps, discharge, or surgery; no changes in breasts. Does not do self-breast exam: "No one ever told me to—am I supposed to?"

SELF-CHECK

1. What would you expect to find for the client in the situation just described?
2. Upon examination, what signs would you expect to find to validate symptoms of your client in Chapter 1?
3. How would you write up your objective findings in SOAP format?
4. How would you approach the examination for each of these clients?

References

1. Jones C: The first gynecological examination: establishing a partnership in health care. *Issues in Health Care of Women* **1**: 3, 1979.
2. Latimis B: Women's health care update. *The Nurse Practitioner* **4**: 40, 1979.
3. Anapol D, Wagner NN: Patient provider preferences and the pelvic examination. *The Nurse Practitioner* **3**: 13, 1978.
4. Tiefer L: A survey of college women's experiences with and attitudes toward pelvic examinations. *Women and Health* **4**: 393, 1979.
5. Taylor D: Contraceptive counseling and care, in Mercer RT: *Perspectives on Adolescent Health Care*. Philadelphia, Lippincott, 1979, p. 139.
6. Miller GD: The gynecological examination as a learning experience. *Journal of the American College Health Association* **23**: 162–164, 1974.
7. Russo NG: Protocol: women's health assessment. *The Nurse Practitioner* **3**: 26, 1978.
8. Gollober M: Screening for cervical cancer, part 1. *The Nurse Practitioner* **4**: 20, 1979.
9. Gollober M: Screening for cervical cancer, part 2. *The Nurse Practitioner* **4**: 18, 1979.

For Further Reading

Bates B: *A Guide to Physical Assessment*, ed 2. Philadelphia, Lippincott, 1979.

Berger K, Fields W: *Pocket Guide to Health Assessment*. Reston, Va, Reston Publishing, 1980.

Gillies DA, Alyn IB: *Patient Assessment and Management by the Nurse Practitioner*. Philadelphia, Saunders, 1976.

Green TH Jr: *Gynecology—Essentials of Clinical Practice*, ed 3. Boston, Little, Brown, 1977.

Martin LL: *Health Care of Women*. Philadelphia, Lippincott, 1978.

McKenzie CAM: Sexuality and the menopausal woman. *Issues in Health Care of Women* **1:** 37–44, 1978.

Patient Assessment: Examination of the Female Pelvis, Part 1 & 2. *American Journal of Nursing* 11, 12, 1–26, 1–28, 1978.

Prior JA, Silberstein JS: *Physical Diagnosis*, ed 5. St. Louis, CV Mosby, 1977.

Sherman JL Jr, Fields SK: *Guide to Patient Evaluation*. Flushing, NY, Medical Examination Publishing, 1974.

Findings

At the end of Chapter 5, you will be able to:

1. describe common findings of the gynecologic examination, normal variations, and characteristics of women at different points of the life span
2. list and describe common aberrations that may be found on vulva and perineum
3. describe causes, symptoms, and observations of vaginal infections
4. describe selected aberrations of the cervix
5. describe selected abnormal findings of ovaries, tubes, uterus, and vagina
6. analyze and evaluate methods of assessment, interventions, and need for referral for each of the selected findings discussed
7. synthesize information in order to write SOAP notes for objective findings, assessment, and plan

In this chapter, normal findings and common aberrations of the woman's reproductive tract are described. Our intention is to present information about those which you may commonly encounter, but we have not included the multiplicity of findings that you may see. The aberrations we have included are appropriate for nursing management and/or initial assessment and screening or are sufficiently common that you may need to recognize them and make a referral. Any lesion, mass, irregularity, or symptom-producing occurrence should be investigated, and if not recognizable by the nurse, a referral should be made. It is essential for nurses practicing in roles as primary care providers to recognize deviations from normal—whether in appearance, palpation, odor, auscultation, or percussion or by subjective symptoms described by the client—and to collaborate with other colleagues on those findings deemed to be outside their realm of expertise. Differential diagnosis most appropriately falls within the scope of medical practice.

Protocols

Protocols can be defined broadly as any standardized format for any or all steps of nursing process, ranging in composition from a formal list to an extensive narrative. There is growing support for use of protocols among legislative mandates. In some states, expanded practice is defined and laws specify use of protocols. In others, the nurse practice act is general. It is important to check the legal scope of practice before designing protocols.[1]

Protocols should be differentiated from standing orders and general guidelines. Protocols include not only guidelines for data collection, but also analysis and a plan. Standing orders often begin with a diagnosis and then tell you what to do as treatment. A number of books of protocols are available that can either be adopted or used as guidelines for development of protocols appropriate for a particular setting (see For Further Reading at the end of the chapter).

Some of the interventions described in this chapter may fall within the scope of nursing management in one state or setting and medical management in another. It is not the intention of this book to provide complete protocols but rather to provide an overview of common findings and interventions and some references for development of appropriate protocols (see an example of a protocol in the Appendix).

Common Aberrations of Vulva and Perineum

Nursing assessment begins with recognition of normal findings and common variations. By sharing findings, you can help reassure the woman of her normalcy. This is particularly important when performing a first pelvic examination or assessing a woman who is experiencing menopausal symptoms. These women are particularly vulnerable to concerns about their normalcy and anatomical integrity as sexual beings.

There is a wide variation in what may be termed normal size and shape of external genitalia in women. Some women have large, long labia majora and protruberant labia minora; others have relatively small labia close to the vaginal opening. It is not unusual for a pair of labia to be unequal in size, that is, one labium majorus larger or longer than the other. In a young adolescent woman who is not yet mature, the labia will be small and firm; with the labia minora hidden by the labia majora. In a woman who has been sexually active and who has had one or more children, the labia will probably be longer and more prominent; the labia minora may be obvious between the labia majora. In an older woman who is postmenopausal, the labia may be atrophic. As fat tissue decreases, tissues of the vulva may become thinner.[2]

Distribution of pubic hair varies markedly from one woman to another. The normal configuration is triangular, with the apex pointing down, but many women have a line of hair extending from mons to umbilicus. Pubic hair may be sparse in women just entering puberty and also in older women as a result of the aging process. A decrease in the amount of fat in the mons may also occur with aging.[3(p197)] The amount and density of hair varies with the individual. Note the amount and distribution of other body hair as a guide in assessment. A very hirsute woman may be perfectly normal or may be experiencing endocrine problems, including Stein-Leventhal, which is associated with infertility. The color of pubic hair is, of course, the result of genetics and will be consistent with other body hair, the exception being whitening as the result of aging.

Atrophy causes skin to be more thin and shiny. Erythema is due to inflammation and may be the result of infection or irritation.[3(p197)] *Candida vaginitis* can cause inflammation and resultant erythema of and between the labia. So can irritation from soap, scented toilet tissue, feminine deodorant hygiene products, and wearing underwear made of synthetic fibers. Check between labia for any accumulation of debris from powder, soap, or hygiene products. Excoriations in a linear pattern result from scratching. Grayish-white, thick plaques may represent leukoplakia and may be cancerous; these should be noted and the woman referred for biopsy.[3(p197)] Leukoplakia is most common in postmenopausal women.

Flat, red, itchy areas ranging from one to several millimeters in diameter and appearing in the groin area and on inner thighs and buttocks may be monilial (yeast) lesions. These may be treated successfully with over-the-counter fungicide creams or liquids. It is particularly important to recognize and treat these lesions and also inquire about the presence of athlete's foot, as the same fungus, *Candida albicans*, causes vaginitis. In women who experience recurrent *Candida vaginitis*, also inquire about presence of such red lesions and athlete's foot in the partner. Treating the partner for superficial groin, buttock, or foot fungus lesions may break the cycle of recurrent *Candida* infections. If the partner is uncircumcised, he may also harbor *Candida* under his foreskin. The symptoms, reddened and often itchy areas, may be treated with over-the-counter fungicide creams, lotions, or sprays.

Skene's and Bartholin's glands may become infected and appear as tender lumps. Symptoms usually include pain, complaints of a lump, and occasionally discharge. If one of these glands appears swollen, attempt to milk the gland for discharge and if present, culture it. To milk the gland, insert index finger in the vagina at area of the duct opening and thumb outside on the labia and apply gentle pressure. You may be able to see the swelling and some erythema and feel enlargement of the gland. Most infections resolve with warm sitz baths and use of antibiotics, when an organism can be identified. If infection exacerbates, persists, or recurs, referral for an incision and drainage may be necessary.[4(p227)]

Warts, also known as venereal warts and condyloma acuminata, appear as raised single or multiple papillary lesions, which sometimes look like cauliflower. They are caused by a virus and range in size from one millimeter to several centimeters in diameter. Symptoms include itching and foul discharge. Warts may be found on the vulva, in the vagina, and around or in the anal area and occasionally on the cervix.

It is important to rule out syphilis, as these organisms mimic condylomata lata, flat, warty growths, which may be a part of second stage syphilis. A gonorrhea culture should also be done. For treatment, swab 25% podophyllin benzoin,[4(p28)] a resin, on lesions and wash off in three to four hours, or earlier if sensation of burning becomes intense. This is a very caustic substance and should be applied carefully to lesions, avoiding surrounding tissue. Repeat treatment weekly until lesions are gone. Self-treatment is not recommended because of the caustic nature of podophyllin.

Treatment may sometimes be the prerogative only of physicians. Medical referral is necessary if there is no response to treatment or if there is recurrence or persistence of lesions. Hygiene measures discussed in Chapter 6 should be suggested to minimize maintenance of moisture. Because warts are common with increased estrogen, it may be necessary to stop oral contraceptives if lesions persist or recur. To avoid contracting the virus and then passing it back, the partner should wear a condom during sex until lesions clear.

The primary stage of syphilis appears 10 to 90 days after exposure as chancres, which are painless lesions varying from a slight erosion to deep ulcerations. Chancres may appear in the same locations as the warts and can also appear on the lips or mucus membranes of the mouth. The painless chancres should be differentiated from the very painful herpes lesions. Chancres that appear on the cervix may escape detection as they may appear as an ectropion. They heal without treatment.

Secondary syphilis presents as skin lesions that are usually bilateral, symmetrical and macular, papular, or papulosquamous. There may be mucous membrane lesions also, lymphadenopathy, fever, and possibly some organ involvement (hepatitis, meningitis). If untreated or unrecognized, these symptoms, too, disappear.[5]

Clients who have contracted syphilis and have never been treated will harbor the *T pallidum* organism in their bodies and have latent syphilis. The dire effects of neurosyphilis demand that we alert our clients to the dangers of the untreated disease and screen all those women who voice any suspicion of exposure. Syphilis is a reportable disease and contacts should be followed up.

To determine if lesions are syphilis or if exposure is suspected or confirmed, a blood test for antibodies is done, either a fluorescent treponemal antibody absorption test (FTA-ABS) or venereal disease research laboratory (VDRL). Penicillin remains the treatment of choice, with follow-up screening for a year at periodic intervals.[4(pp276–277)] One year with negative serologic tests is necessary for a cure to be pronounced.

Tender, painful blister-like lesions on labia, introitus, or perineum are probably herpes virus 2. They are characterized by the pain they cause, and they may also be itchy. Fever, malaise, pain on urination, and regional adenopathy may also occur. Lesions may excoriate and crust over. Because the lesions are similar to chancres of syphilis, a dark-field exam or blood antibody test should be done. Lesions may last up to six weeks and are often recurrent at varying intervals.[6(pp87–88)]

Interventions are symptomatic at present and include using of analgesics, sitz baths, bacitracin or Betadine Scrub on lesions, camphor, alcohol, topical xylocaine, cool wet tea bags; flushing genitalia with cool water after urinating; keeping vulva dry; wearing cotton underclothing; and offering much reassurance. A recent study holds some promise for miconazale nitrate 2% (Monistat®) for relief of symptoms and diminution of recurrence.[7] Women with recurrent herpes should have Pap smears every six months, as there seems to be some relationship between herpes infections and cervical cancer. The woman should abstain or have her partner use condoms when lesions are present.

Pediculosis pubis, infestation with pubic lice, may occur through direct contact or contact with clothing, towels, bedding, furniture, or toilet seats. Commonly called crabs, these parasites can be seen as tiny black or brown flecks. The most common symptom is itching. There may also be nits (eggs) in hair shafts. Interventions include using shampoo specific for lice, a fine-toothed combing to remove nits, laundering of bedding and clothes, and using spray or bug bomb for nonlaunderable items such as mattresses and pillows. Crabs live only about 24 hours off a warm body, but eggs live approximately six days.[8(p114),9(p61)]

Molluscum contagiosum is a viral infection spread by direct contact that causes fleshy papular umbilicated skin-colored lesions one to 15 mm on genitalia. They may resemble condyloma acuminata, but are unresponsive to podophyllin. These lesions are not painful or itchy. Referral to a physician is necessary as excision is treatment of choice. The lesion may be identified with Wright's, Giemsa, or gram stain.[10(p34)]

Chancroid is caused by a bacillus, is spread sexually, and appears as soft maculopapular lesions on external genitalia. These lesions are painful and tender and characterized by profuse foul discharge. There may be adenopathy or erythema. A dark-field exam as well as a VDRL should be done to rule out syphilis. A gonorrhea culture and gram stain should also be done. Treatment is antibiotic-specific, tetracycline, streptomycin, or sulfanomides and follow-up. Referral for aspiration or incision and drainage may be necessary.[4(p277),10(p37)]

Granuloma inguinale is caused by bacteria and spread sexually. It causes small, circumscribed, elevated lesions on vulva, vagina, or perineum that may have foul discharge. Giemsa and Wright's stain, VDRL, and gonorrhea culture should be done. Intervention is tetracycline or streptomycin. If no interventions occur, the condition becomes chronic and causes ulceration of genitalia resembling cancer.[8(pp110–111),10(p38),4(pp278–279)]

Elephantiasis of vulva occurs with sexually acquired lymphogranuloma venereum, caused by a filterable virus, along with systemic symptoms of infection. There is marked adenopathy of entire region and deep necrosis and ulcerations can occur without interventions. The Frei test should be done, as well as VDRL. Selected antibiotics are used for treatment.[4(pp277–278)]

Any lesions should be treated as abnormal and either diagnosed and treated or referred. Carcinoma of the vulva does occur, so strange lesions should be suspect and prompt medical referral made.

Vaginal Findings and Common Infections

The introitus in a young woman may be very small or tight with a small hymenal opening. If the hymen is imperforate, referral must be made so that an opening can be created. A woman who is sexually active and one who has had one or more children will have hymenal tags or remnants present. She may also have evidence of a median or mediolateral episiotomy on the perineum, although the area should be intact and well healed.

Women who have had children and older women may have a cystocele, urethrocele, or rectocele present due to relaxation of pelvic soft tissues. Bulging in the anterior wall indicates a cystocele or urethrocele; in the posterior wall, a rectocele.[3(p197)]

The urethra may be reddened or appear irritated. Milk it and culture any discharge. Irritation of the meatus is common in older postmenopausal women due to diminution of estrogen and atrophy of tissues. Cautious use of estrogen creams may help.

The vaginal vault may be atrophic in older women, pink and velvety in appearance.[2] Absence of rugae is indicative of diminishing estrogen levels.[3(p197)]

Erythema and edema along with profuse or foul-smelling discharge are characteristic of vaginitis. Discharge that is blood-streaked, serosanguineous, thin to thick, scanty to profuse, grayish, and foul-smelling may indicate presence of a foreign body. Young children often put objects in their vaginas. Menstruating women sometimes forget a tampon, or the tampon shreds and disintegrates. The foreign body may also be a condom or diaphragm or clumps of pubic hair pulled in during intercourse.[11(p227)] If it looks like a secondary infection may be present, culture the discharge.

Vaginal discharge due to allergy or irritation reaction to soaps, deodorant tampons, feminine hygiene products, condoms, and contraceptive creams, jellies, or foams and so on cannot be characterized easily. A careful history will aid in assessment, and smears to rule out *Trichomoniasis* and *Candida* should be done to rule out infection secondary to irritation. Ruling out and eliminating possible irritants will confirm the diagnosis.[11(p227)]

The appearance of lining, bleeding, inflammation, friability of vaginal wall, any lesions seen or felt, cysts, tumors, cystocele, or rectocele should all be referred for treatment. Condyloma may appear on the vaginal wall.

Organisms that may be cultured from the vaginas of women experiencing no symptoms include *lactobacillus* (normal bacterial flora), *Staphylococcus aureus* and *albus*, *Escherichia coli*, *Proteus*, *Streptococcus*, and *Mycoplasma*. Any of the latter six of these can also be implicated as symptom-producing.

Trichomoniasis, caused by a protozoan, and yeast (monilia) infections, caused by *Candida albicans*, are the most common vaginal infections women present with. *Trichomonas vaginalis* infection is characterized by watery, frothy, foul, yellowish-green-gray discharge; pain; itching; and burning. The cervix may be red and is characterized as a "strawberry cervix." There may be dyspareunia and burning on urination or following intercourse. This infection may be responsible for a Class II Pap smear. A gonorrhea culture should be done, as well as urinalysis and an NaCl wet smear.[10(p28),6(pp86–87)]

Interventions include Flagyl® (metronidazole) for woman and partner, abstinence during therapy, and a recheck after a week of treatment. In addition to side effects such as nausea, vomiting, headache, and abdominal distress when alcoholic beverages are consumed, some concern has been expressed about the dangers of Flagyl. Its safety in pregnancy has not been demonstrated.[12,13] Teaching about hygiene measures to prevent recurrence is important (see Chapter 6).

Candida is recognized by a cottage cheese-like, white, odorless discharge that causes pain, itching, erythema, and burning on urination. Intercourse may be painful. Diagnosis is based on clinical assessment and wet smear or KOH slide mount. The spores or hyphae of *Candida* can sometimes be seen on a wet prep slide.

Vaginal suppositories or cream of nystatin are used for therapy. It is important to assess carefully for precipitating factors: diabetes and poor dietary habits seem to provide a favorable milieu for yeast. Use of oral contraceptives, pregnancy, oral or anal sex, generally lowered resistance, and oral use of antibiotics that suppress natural bacteria all seem to contribute. So does failure to adhere to the hygiene measures described in Chapter 6. If discharge is severe, a vinegar douche at the outset may help, but douching should not be repeated. Cortisone creams applied to vulva and perineum help to relieve symptoms, as will sitz baths.[10(p27),6(pp 85–86)] Creams containing cortisone should not be used more than four days, however, due to systemic absorption.

Hemophilus vaginalis or nonspecific vaginitis is caused by corynebacterium vaginale or hemophilus vaginalis and is related to allergies to soaps, tight clothing, rectal intercourse, and poor lubrication. On a wet prep slide, the epithelial cells appear stippled due to adherence of bacteria. These are called clue cells. Symptoms are itching and grayish discharge, with some odor, usually fishy or musty. If bacteria are present, a sulfa vaginal cream may help. The FDA has raised a query as to the effectiveness of sulfa vaginal creams in the treatment of hemophilus vaginalis. Although the product relieves symptoms, it does not seem effective against the organism. A triple sulfonamide preparation was demonstrated to be effective in one study. Further investigations are under way at present.[14] When allergies to sulfa preclude its use, try acijel or other creams or gels designed to restore pH and natural flora.[4(p235)] Attention to hygiene, soaps, and so on also helps (see Chapter 6).

Gonorrhea (also called clap or drip) is usually symptomless in women, but may produce vaginal discharge, urinary tract symptoms, and/or pelvic pain. Incubation is 3 to 30 days. Skene's or Bartholin's glands may be inflamed, discharge is often creamy yellow, and the cervix may appear erythematous. The woman may also have gonococcal pharyngitis. It is wise to screen for urinary tract infections, as well as to do cultures. Cervical, anal, and nasopharyngeal cultures should be done. Treatment is penicillin, usually preceded by benemid for absorption, and follow-up for cultures until negative.[4(p247)] To avoid spread, all contacts should be cultured and treated. Males usually report symptoms of urethritis and a thick yellow discharge. Gonorrhea is a reportable communicable disease so appropriate forms must be completed and contacts followed up.

Chlamydia trachomatis, an intracellular parasite, has been implicated as the cause of more vaginal infections in college-age women than has gonorrhea. The woman may be symptomless, but pass the organism to her partner, who may then develop urethritis or epididymytis. Symptoms for the woman, when they occur, include vaginal discharge and sometimes urethritis and signs of pelvic inflammatory disease. Cultures, if positive, should require treatment with tetracycline or erythromycin.[15,16]

T Mycoplasma and *Mycoplasma hominis* can also cause vaginitis and have been implicated in causing infertility and spontaneous abortion.[3(p377)] In the presence of persistent symptoms, when smears are negative for *Trichomonas* and *Candida*, hygiene is attended to, and gonorrhea ruled out, *Mycoplasma* should be suspected. This organism can be cultured in the laboratory. The treatment of choice is tetracycline or demeclocycline.

Atrophic vaginitis may occur in women past menopause due to lack of estrogen. Burning, irritation, itching, pain on intercourse, lack of lubrication, and bladder symptoms are common. Irritation around the urinary meatus may be seen. Use of estrogen cream may clear the symptoms. It is important to rule out carcinoma, to discuss hygiene, and to talk with the woman who is sexually active to help her understand that adequate lubrication is necessary. Longer foreplay, use of saliva, or water-soluble jelly lubricants all will help. Because estrogen cream can be absorbed systemically, it should be reserved for cautious use with the informed consent of the woman for as brief a time as possible to relieve symptoms.[11(pp212–213)]

Cervix

Common findings of the cervix include polyps, nabothian cysts, cervicitis, ectropion, and, less commonly, tears or scars. It should be noted that condyloma and herpes virus type 2 lesions can also appear on the cervix. Tears and scars should be described as to extent and location and referred for evaluation if they appear to be bleeding or infected or give cause for suspicion of need for interventions.

A polyp appears as a nubbin of tissue usually protruding from the os; it is often cherry red (see Figure 5.1). It may cause irregular bleeding or postmenstrual bleeding. Referral is necessary for excision.

Nabothian cysts are plugged mucus gland ducts on the cervix that appear as yellow or orangish blobs on the surface of the cervix (see Figure 5.2). There are no interventions specific to these.[11(pp336–337)]

Ectropion, also known as cervical erosion, is the result of extension of columnar epithelium onto the surface of the cervix beyond the endocervical canal. The borders are usually regular (see Figure 5.3). About 15 to 20% of women exhibit an ectropion. The appearance of the cervix is attributable to visibility of the junction between squamous and the more vascular columnar epithelium. It is important to check regularly for symptoms and to culture for organisms if there is chronic vaginal discharge. An ectropion may be responsible for a Class II Pap. If extensive or friable, referral for cryosurgery or electrocautery is necessary. Some-

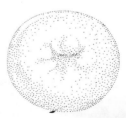

Figure 5.1   Cervical Polyp

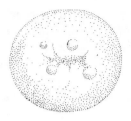

Figure 5.2   Nabothian Cyst

times a colposcopy or punch biopsy may be indicated.[10(pp32-33)] Cervical carcinoma is often granular and friable and has irregular borders.

A true cervicitis may arise involving an extensive area of the cervix and appearing as a red, friable, and often bleeding and irritated cervix. Interventions are aimed at identifying any organism present, careful screening for carcinoma, and often referral for appropriate treatment, such as cryosurgery or cautery to restore normal epithelium.[4(pp240-241)]

A hooded appearance of the cervix is characteristic of women exposed in utero to DES (diethylstilbestrol). For all women so exposed or suspected of exposure, referral should be made for further evaluations such as Schiller's test, biopsy, and/or colposcopy. Ectropion are also common in these women.[4(pp128-132)]

If the woman has an IUD in place, you should be able to see the strings. If you encounter something hard in the os during the bimanual exam, it may be the IUD, which is displaced.

The Pap smear is a screening for carcinoma of the cervix and vagina. Classes of Pap smears are as follows:

Class I: benign
Class II: atypical, not suspicious for cancer
Class III: atypical, suspicious for cancer
Class IV: probable cancer cells
Class V: carcinoma in situ

Classes II and III may result from extensive ectropion, cervicitis, and/or chronic vaginitis. It is important, therefore, to screen for infections, assess carefully for cause, and treat or refer for treatment and evaluation and repeat the Pap smear. Some protocols suggest referral for colposcopy for every Class III smear. Also some suggest a Schiller's test and repeat Pap smears for Class II at the same time in menstrual cycle as the first one after treatment of any infection. Lab reports may include indication of estrogen effect due to timing of cycle, oral contraceptives, pregnancy, or estrogen replacement therapy post-menopause.[6(pp96-98),10 (p45)]

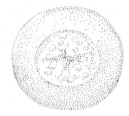

Figure 5.3 Ectropion

Ovaries

The ovaries of a woman after menopause are usually smaller than those in a menstruating woman and should not be tender.[3(p201)] Most common aberrations of ovaries are cysts and tumors. These are generally detected as masses in adnexa or as irregularities of menses, amenorrhea, prolonged flow, pelvic pain, and hemorrhage if they rupture. Any irregularity, enlargement, or mass in adnexa, whether or not accompanied by symptoms, should be referred for further evaluation.

Tubes

Fallopian tubes may be the site of ectopic pregnancy, cysts, tumors, or infections. In an older woman, a cystic and hard tube is characteristic of carcinoma. A sausage-shaped tube indicates pelvic inflammation.[3(p201)] There may be serous or bloody vaginal discharge. Hemorrhage and shock can occur if an ectopic pregnancy ruptures the tube. Adnexal mass, a large palpable tube, pelvic pain or discomfort, persistent dull aching, and low-grade temperature are all suspicious and referral should be made.

Uterus

Pregnancy causes enlargement of the uterus and softening of the juncture between cervix and corpus. It is important to rule out pregnancy by history and laboratory test, as well as pelvic examination. Fibroid tumors of the uterus may appear as irregular masses and cause enlargement, as may other types of benign and malignant tumors. Irregular menses or postmenstrual bleeding are common clinical symptoms. Crampy pain may also be present, and, if tumors are large enough, pressure on other organs. Any enlargement of the uterus, irregularity in configuration, nodular masses, change in contours, pain, or unusual bleeding are all cause for referral for further evaluation.

The nonpregnant uterus before menopause is usually the size of a small fist. After menopause, it is even smaller. Displacement or lack of mobility may indicate pelvic tumor or adhesions.

Prolapse of the uterus should be checked for and referred. Prolapse is due to relaxation of supporting ligaments and muscles of the pelvic floor. Prolapse may be evident on inspection or palpation, as well as by history of symptoms. Women who have a prolapse should be advised not to jog until the uterus can be repaired.

PID

Pelvic inflammatory disease (PID) may result from viral or bacterial infection of tubes, uterus, ovaries, pelvic vessels, and lymphatics, and/or peritoneal cavity. The most common organism is *N gonorrhoeae*. It has been estimated that 10 to 17% of women who have gonorrhea develop PID.[17] Other organisms implicated include peptostreptococci and bacteroides species, *Escherichia coli, Mycoplasma hominis,* and *Chlamydia trachomatis.*[18] Symptoms include pain, low-grade fever, malaise, and sometimes nausea and vomiting. Vaginal discharge may increase and may be foul-smelling. On examination, the areas affected will be tender and painful and adnexa may be swollen and tender. Touching the cervix will cause pain, known as Chandelier's sign. Assessments include screening to rule out urinary tract involvement, pregnancy test, cultures for organism including *N gonorrhoeae*, a CBC (WBC and sedimentation rate may be elevated), VDRL, and referral to rule out other causes. Referral for treatment—which includes bedrest, possible hospitalization, appropriate antibiotics, analgesics, and general support—is necessary.[6(pp99–100),10(pp31–32)]

Toxic-Shock Syndrome

Toxic-shock syndrome was first described as a distinct entity in 1978. Although the age range is 13 to 52, it is confined mostly to women under 30 and is characterized by sudden onset of high fever, vomiting and diarrhea, and eventual severe prolonged shock and hypotension.[19,20] The organism implicated thus far is *Staphylococcus aureus*. Often an erythematous macular desquamating rash is present, notably on palms and soles. The fatality rate is 3 to 10%.[21]

Evidence continues to accumulate implicating tampons as possible culture media for bacteria or acting to promote release or absorption of toxin from the vagina into the bloodstream.[22] Tampons designed as mesh bags containing tiny synthetic sponges have been implicated twice as often in toxic-shock cases as those of the more conventional, tubular cottonoid design.[20] One brand of tampon has been withdrawn from the market due to association with occurrence of toxic-shock syndrome.

As a result of the more than 100 new cases reported between January and July of 1980, women who wish to reduce the small risk of toxic shock have been advised to use tampons when needed for heavy flow and not for the entire menses or for 24 hours at a time. Those who have survived toxic shock should use no tampons until eradication of *S aureus* is accomplished.

Treatment of women affected is based on support of massive fluid and electrolyte needs, therapy with a beta-lactamase-resistant antibiotic after obtaining cultures, and supportive intervention for shock.[10] The primary care nurse needs to be aware of symptoms in order to recognize toxic shock as early as possible and refer the woman for prompt intervention.

Dysmenorrhea

Dysmenorrhea is a common complaint of premenopausal women. It may be either primary, therefore unrelated to pathology, or secondary to establishment of a comfortable pattern of menses. It is generally thought to be related to sensitivity of the uterus, contractions designed to expel the endometrial lining or menstrual flow, the role of prostaglandins not yet fully understood,[23] and torsion on the ligaments that suspend the uterus. Any complaint of severe or disabling cramps should be investigated to rule out anatomical aberration and causative pathology. Referral should always be made for any woman desiring it and for any suggestion of pathology.

Every effort should be made to provide for comfort measures for women who suffer if no treatable pathology or anomaly is found. Warm baths, a heating pad or hot water bottle, analgesics, exercise, attention to avoidance of fluid retention, and good bowel hygiene all may help. Intercourse with orgasm will alleviate or diminish cramps in some women. Ibuprofen (Motrin), which inhibits prostaglandin synthesis, has been found to be of help in treating primary dysmenorrhea.[24] So has use of mefenamic acid (Ponstel), which has been demonstrated to inhibit prostaglandin synthesis and activity.[25] Referral for assessment and possible prescription of one of these should be considered in cases of severe primary dysmenorrhea in the absence of pathology when other relief measures are of little or no use.

Irregular Bleeding

Bleeding after menopause may have several origins. It may be the result of the menstrual irregularities that herald menopause, whereby after several months of amenorrhea, menses resume, or it may be due to pathology. Once menopause is established with at least a year of amenorrhea, suspicion should be focused on carcinoma. Any woman with vaginal bleeding should have a complete gynecological examination and Pap smear. Some physicians deem it prudent to do an endometrial biopsy or dilation and curretage to rule out carcinoma and to establish cause. A number of drugs may also cause bleeding, including phenothiazines, anticholinergics, anticoagulants, thiazides, and diuretics.

Vaginal bleeding before menarche may be the result of several causes. By careful history and physical assessment, the practitioner needs to rule out presence of a foreign body in the vagina, pregnancy, improper use of oral contraceptives, tumor, vaginitis, DES exposure, and blood dyscrasias.

Bladder and Urethra

Cystitis is a common occurrence in women due to the short relatively straight urethra and the close proximity of the anal area and *Escherichia coli*. Symptoms include pain and burning on urination, frequency, urgency, hesitancy, and blood in the urine.[26(p8)] It is important to differentiate between cystitis and vaginitis and to rule out each in the presence of the other when symptoms for both are present. Virtually all cases of cystitis occurring in the well, ambulatory population are caused by *E coli*.

A clean voided specimen is best for diagnosis. The woman should be instructed to wash her labia and then spread her labia and collect a midstream specimen in a sterile container. Soap should not be used to wash, as residues will kill bacteria.

Characteristics of urine include pH (normally 4.8–7.8), specific gravity (normal 1.002–1.030), and glucose, albumin, and occult blood (all normally absent). Presence of bacteria in numbers greater than 10^5 per milliliter indicates infection. Epithelial cells and white blood cells are also indicative of cystitis. Casts are present only when there is renal involvement.

Urine may also be cultured. Prompt refrigeration (within ten to 15 minutes) after collection is necessary for an accurate culture.

Treatment may be instituted with sulfonamides or ampicillin if allergy to sulfa exists. Phenazopyridine HC1 may be used for bladder analgesia, 100 mg every six hours for two or three days. This will color the urine orange.[10(pp47–48)] Some practitioners discourage its use as it masks symptoms and may delay institution of proper antibacterial therapy. It also gives a false impression of cure and women may stop antibacterial medication before completing full course of treatment.

Some women also experience chronic urethritis as a result of the location and anatomy of the urethra. Infection or irritation is common. If discharge can be milked from the urethra and bacteria can be cultured, appropriate antibacterials can be used. For irritation, identify irritants— such as soaps, deodorant hygiene and menstrual care products, tight clothing, soap or fabric softener residues in clothing, colored and scented toilet tissue—discontinue their use, and follow up. If urethritis seems to be related to sexual activity, alternative positions and adequate foreplay and lubrication may be suggested. Voiding after intercourse will flush bacteria from the urethra and help to prevent *E coli* infection carried from the nearby anal area during penile thrusting. Referral for more aggressive medical management may be necessary if symptoms are persistent and uncomfortable, and no relief occurs with noninvasive care.[27]

Summary

In assessment, it is important to recognize the normal and to further evaluate and refer for any deviations. It should be noted that many of the sexually transmitted diseases such as herpes virus type 2, syphilis, and gonorrhea have serious effects on pregnancy. Likewise, treatments such as certain medications may be harmful to a pregnancy. It is prudent, therefore, to be assured that pregnancy is not a possibility before treatment is instituted. If the woman is pregnant, risks to her fetus need to be evaluated and explained carefully so she can decide whether to continue the pregnancy.

Sample Write-up for Pelvic Examination

The following are findings for Marie Valdarez, the client described in Chapter 4.

Subjective: "My last Pap smear was a couple of years ago, and I think I should have one. Also, it is painful to have sex, and it itches 'down there'. It burns, too, when urine comes out. Sometimes I lose urine (small amount) when I cough." Denies blood in urine, bladder spasms, frequency. States she wears underwear to bed, uses bubble bath occasionally and baby powder daily. Had a hysterectomy in 1968—"They took out everything."

Objective: Vulva appears atrophied; erythema noted around meatus; some erythema and caked deposit between labia; no lesions noted; perineum clean, no lesions; anal area, no lesions, fissures, erythema, or hemorrhoids. Vaginal walls appear thin, atrophied, pale pink in color; no lesions noted and no irregularities.

Bimanual exam: uterus and cervix absent; no masses or tenderness in adnexa; slight cystocele palpated when client bears down.

Rectal exam: negative—no masses felt, rectovaginal wall intact, no rectocele.

SELF-CHECK

1. What findings would you expect for your client in Chapter 1? For the client in Chapter 4?
2. Continue SOAP notes for the client in Chapter 1.
3. What would your assessment be for the clients in Chapters 1 and 4?
4. How would you validate your assessments?
5. Write up assessments as part of your SOAP notes and write your plan.
6. Make a problem list for each of these clients.

References

1. Pearson LB: Protocols: how to develop and implement within the nurse practitioner's setting. *Nurse Practitioner* 1: 9–11, 1976.
2. McKenzie CAM: Sexuality and the menopausal woman. *Issues in Health Care of Women* 1: 39, 1978.
3. Futrell M, Brovender S, McKinnon-Mullett E, et al: *Primary Health Care of the Older Adult*. North Scituate, Mass, Duxbury Press, 1980.
4. Green TH Jr: *Gynecology—Essentials of Clinical Practice*, ed 3. Boston, Little, Brown, 1977.
5. *Criteria and Techniques for the Diagnosis of Early Syphilis*. Atlanta, Center for Disease Control, 1978.
6. Martin LL: Gynecological problems, in Bullough B (ed) *The Management of Common Human Miseries*. New York, Springer, 1979.
7. Blough HA, Giuntoli RL: Successful treatment of human genital herpes infections with 2-deoxy-D-glucose. *Journal of the American Medical Association* 241: 2798–2801, 1979.
8. Chiappa JA, Forish JJ: *The VD Book*. New York, Holt Rinehart & Winston, 1977.
9. Schwartz L: Common skin problems, in Bullough B (ed) *The Management of Common Human Miseries*. New York, Springer, 1979.
10. Gyn Family Planning Nurse Practitioners: *A Manual of Standard Practice Procedures and Policies*. Storrs, Conn, University of Connecticut Women's Health Clinic, 1980.
11. Martin LL: *Health Care of Women*. Philadelphia, Lippincott, 1978.
12. *Talk Paper*, T75-73. Rockville, Md, US Dept of Health, Education and Welfare, Public Health Service, Food and Drug Administration, 1975, pp 1–2.
13. Weltman R: New metronidazole study: same reassuring findings for now. *Journal of the American Medical Association*. 239: 1371, 1978.
14. Sulfa vaginal creams. *FDA Drug Bulletin* 10: 6, 1980.
15. McCormach WM, et al: Fifteen-month follow-up study of women infected with Chlamydia trachomatis. *New England Journal of Medicine* 300: 123–125, 1979.

16. Ridenour N: Chlamydia. *The Nurse Practitioner* **5:** 45, 48, 1980.
17. Eschenbach DA, Holmes KK: Acute pelvic inflammatory disease: current concepts of pathogenesis, etiology, and management. *Clinical Obstetrics and Gynecology* **18:** 35, 1975.
18. Thompson SE, Hager WD: Acute pelvic inflammatory disease. *Sexually Transmitted Diseases* **4:** 107, 1977.
19. Toxic-shock cases: a staph syndrome? *Science News* **117:** 343, 1980.
20. Toxic-shock culprits. *Science News* **118:** 198, 1980.
21. Advisory on toxic-shock syndrome. *FDA Drug Bulletin* **10:** 10–11, 1980.
22. Toxic shock linked to use of tampons. *Science News* **118:** 6, 1980.
23. Cures for Cramps. *Science News* **116:** 22, 1979.
24. Drugs for dysmenorrhea. *Medical Letters Drugs Therapy* **21:** 81, 1979.
25. Budoff PW: Use of mefenamic acid in the treatment of primary dysmenorrhea. *Journal of the American Medical Association* **241:** 2713–2716, 1979.
26. Schwarz H: *Urinary Tract Infections.* Norwich, NY, Norwich-Eaton Pharmaceuticals.
27. Pilmer GA: *Chronic Urethritis in the Female.* Norwich, NY, Norwich-Eaton Pharmaceuticals, 1963.

For Further Reading

Brown, LK: Toxic shock syndrome. *The American Journal of Maternal Child Nursing* **6:** 57–59, 1981.
Bullough B (ed): *The Management of Common Human Miseries.* New York, Springer, 1979.
Gollober M: Screening for cervical cancer, part 1. *The Nurse Practitioner* **4:** 20–24, 31, 1979.
Gollober M: Screening for cervical cancer, part 2. *The Nurse Practitioner* **4:** 17–18, 1979.
Hoole AH, Greenberg RA, Pickard CC: *Patient Care Guidelines for Family Nurse Practitioners.* Boston, Little, Brown, 1976.
Hudak CM, Redstone PM, Hokanson NC, Suzuki IE: *Clinical Protocols: A Guide for Nurses and Physicians.* Philadelphia, Lippincott, 1976.
Jones C: The first gynecological examination: establishing a partnership in health care. *Issues in Health Care of Women* **1:** 6, 1979.
Klaus BJ: *Protocols Handbook for Nurse Practitioners.* New York, Wiley, 1979.
Rafferty, EG: Chlamydial infections in women. *Journal of Obstetric, Gynecologic and Neonatal Nursing* **10:** 299–301, 1981.
Russo NG: Protocol: women's health assessment. *The Nurse Practitioner* **3:** 23–26, 43, 1978.
Siegel MA, Bullough B: Constructing and adopting protocols. *American Journal of Nursing* **10:** 1616–1618, 1977.
Wrobleski, SS: Toxic shock syndrome. *American Journal of Nursing* **81:** 82–85, 1981.

Primary Prevention and Intervention

At the end of Chapter 6, you will be able to:

1. analyze self-care practices that contribute to promulgation of infections
2. develop teaching and management protocols for clients concerning hygiene and personal care that help to prevent vaginal infections and irritations
3. synthesize previous learning about nutrition for teaching about primary prevention in relation to health of reproductive organs
4. plan management strategies for sexually active women for common problems in intercourse: pain, infection, and contraception

Self-Care Practices

Increasingly, women are assuming control over their bodies and are demanding information for self-care. The advertising industry has attempted to convince women that they need vaginal douche and deodorant products, and manufacturers have scented and deodorized any number of menstrual and self-care products, ranging from tampons and sanitary napkins to toilet tissue and bath soaps. Women have indicated appreciation of learning about self-care procedures during pelvic examinations.

Teaching about self-care practices and products is an important part of primary health care for women. Women providers can be particularly sensitive and understanding toward women who are clients.

A number of self-care practices contribute to occurrence of vaginitis, increased discharge, and irritation of the vulva and perineum. Teaching is an important component of primary care and prevention of problems as well as prevention of recurrence when infections and irritations do arise.

Douching, once a common hygienic practice also considered to be a method of contraception, contributes to vaginitis in a number of ways. Solutions used may alter the pH of the vagina, making it more receptive to organisms that cause infections by suppressing the growth of normal flora. Solutions, too, may be irritating to the vaginal mucosa. If douching is done improperly under too much pressure, the solution may be forced into the uterus and cause irritation or infection. Caustic solutions have been known to cause scarring of the vaginal mucosa and cervix. The perfumes or deodorants used in commerical douching products can be irritants to the sensitive vaginal mucosa.

Douching should be confined to such therapeutic uses as restoring normal pH. It is not a safe method of contraception, as sperm may enter the cervix 60 to 90 seconds after ejaculation occurs.

Baths or showers are the most important means of assuring prevention of infection, removal of secretions, and elimination of undesirable odors. Vaginal deodorant sprays are expensive substitutes for soap and water and may cause itching and rashes in some women. The method of

71

washing may, however, be implicated in causing irritation or increasing susceptibility to infection. Washing of pubic hair and around the anal area with soap is necessary to remove secretions and residue from elimination. It is pubic hair and not skin that harbors odors.

Removal of body hair is a personal decision, but women may ask advice or present with symptoms related to shaving, use of depilatories, or commercial hair removal techniques. The woman who has had treatments to remove hair around her areola may experience inflammation or infection of the hair follicle, resulting in pain, tenderness, formation of a palpable lump, and erythema. This same phenomenon may occur when hair removal is attempted on any part of the body. Axillary or groin nodes may enlarge and become tender secondary to trauma caused by shaving axilla and pubic areas. The removal of a significant portion of pubic hair covering the mons and labia may result in symptoms of irritation; appearance of a rash; and complaints of labial, clitoral, vaginal, and/or urethral soreness, irritation, or itching. Hair, although it can harbor odors and organisms, also performs a protective function. A careful history will help to sort out relationships between onset of symptoms and hair removal.

Washing between labia and around the vaginal introitus with soap removes normal bacteria and also can be very irritating. This practice may cause itching, increased discharge, and a rash. Deodorant soaps are particularly irritating. Thorough rinsing with warm water while labia are separated gently is sufficient to remove secretions.

It should be noted that vaginal discharge is normal, and variations are expected in relation to timing of the menstrual cycle, pregnancy, onset of menopause, and extent of sexual activity. Women who begin using a diaphragm with contraceptive jelly or cream, contraceptive foam, or suppositories or who are sexually active for the first time will experience increased discharge of a new character as the result of the contraceptive products and semen. Normal discharge smells relatively earthy or like menses and becomes thicker and more profuse at and after ovulation, being more watery and less tenacious in the first part of the cycle. It should be clear to slightly mucoid-whitish in color. After intercourse, it will, of course, be mixed with semen. Some women dislike the feeling of semen and douche to remove it. The woman's body will discharge it naturally; removal may be hastened by washing with warm water and inserting a finger in the vagina, rotating it quickly in a spiral motion and removing the most tenacious of the ejaculate.

Women should be taught from the time they are very young to wipe from front to back after elimination, to apply sanitary napkins and mini pads from front to back, and to insert tampons carefully to avoid contaminating them around the anal area. The woman's urethra is short and *Escherichia coli*, which normally reside in the bowel, are principal causes of cystitis. Urinating frequently also helps to prevent infections, as bacteria multiply rapidly in urine when there is stasis. Urinating before insertion of a diaphragm and before and when it is comfortable after intercourse will help to prevent stasis and wash out any bacteria carried into the urethra.

Urinating frequently will also help the woman to avoid bouts of cystitis since bacteria multiply rapidly when there is urinary stasis. Bladder hygiene includes regular and complete emptying of the bladder. Good bladder tone can be maintained by performing pelvic floor (Kegel) exercises. Instruct the woman to stop and start the flow of urine several times when she urinates. Once conscious control of the perivaginal and periurethral muscles is attained, these exercises of tightening and relaxing the pelvic floor muscles can be performed several times a day. They are also beneficial for women who experience relaxation of the pelvic floor structures and resultant stress incontinence or lack of control.

Scented and colored toilet tissues can be very irritating and should be eliminated if symptoms occur. Reports of burning, itching, rash, and chronic feelings of irritation have been given by women (and men) using these products.

Soaps that are heavily perfumed may cause erythema, itching, and rashes when used on the vulva and perineum. So can vaginal deodorant sprays, notorious for causing irritations and allergic responses. Talcum powders may contain perfumes and metallic talc, both of which may be irritating. Talcum powders also tend to cake between the labia and can irritate the meatus. Cornstarch may be used as a safe substitute and is available in shaker cans, as well as in the conventional bulk pack kitchen form.

Tampons and sanitary pads are now perfumed, scented, or deodorized by some manufacturers. These are often implicated in causing irritation, erythema, discharge, and itching and also in contributing to infection by suppressing normal bacteria. Some tampons shred easily and fragments may be left behind in the vagina when the tampon is removed. These fragments provide a medium for growth of organisms and may also cause foul-smelling vaginal discharge. Women should be advised that this can occur and to change the brand of tampons if they find theirs shredding and disintegrating. The filler products for tampons have been considered proprietary secrets. Recently one brand containing small synthetic sponges was removed from the market after being implicated in relation to toxic-shock syndrome.

Some women choose to use pieces of natural sponges to collect men-

strual flow and then wash and reuse them. They feel this is a safer practice than the perils of unknown fillers used in commercial tampons.
Menstrual cups made of plastic are also available to collect the flow, or a
diaphragm may be used. Some women's self-help groups practice menstrual extraction using a sterile cannula and large plastic syringe to suck
out the endometrial lining. This technique is also used for early abortions. It should be performed only by an experienced practitioner using
sterile equipment to avoid infection and great caution to avoid perforation of the uterus.

Clothing

Wearing underwear to bed can contribute to the occurrence of infection,
irritation, and increased vaginal discharge. The vulva, perineum, and
vaginal area have very active glands. Underwear worn to bed, clothing
and underwear of synthetic fabrics, and pantyhose, especially worn under slacks, cause moisture to accumulate. Most organisms implicated as
agents causing vaginitis thrive in dark, warm, moist environments, notably *Trichomonas* and *Candida*, as well as condyloma and herpes virus.
Encourage women to wear garments of cotton, to wear skirts, not to
wear pantyhose (especially under slacks), to choose pantyhose with a
cotton crotch, and not to wear underwear to bed.

Products used to launder garments may contribute to infection and
cause irritation, rash, increased discharge, and allergic responses. Laundry soaps should be measured and clothes rinsed well to remove soap
residues. Powdered detergents often have sawdust fillers that permeate
clothes and are difficult to remove. Fabric softeners are irritants responsible for many rashes. Laundry soaps can also suppress normal vaginal
bacterial flora if they are present as residues in clothing, particularly in
underwear.

Diet

Roughage and sufficient fluids are necessary to promote good bladder
and bowel hygiene. Women who experience chronic constipation may
find intercourse uncomfortable due to the proximity of bowel and vagina. In addition, they will be poor candidates for using a diaphragm, as
hard fecal material will distort the vagina and cause pressure against the
diaphragm when it is in place. Whole grain products, unprocessed bran,
fresh and dried fruit, fresh vegetables high in fiber, seeds and nuts, at
least six to eight glasses of liquid per day, and avoidance of highly refined

or processed foods all contribute to good bowel hygiene. A diet assessment that takes into account cultural traditions, likes and dislikes, and food habits will help you to plan, with the woman, an individualized dietary regime to intervene with this problem. Adequate fluid intake also helps to prevent cystitis. Cranberry juice helps to keep urine acidic, which prevents infection, as does vitamin C.

A diet high in carbohydrates appears to contribute to occurrence of vaginitis, particularly Candida, by providing an environment high in sugar, which is necessary for yeasts to multiply. Women who have recurrent yeast infections should have a fasting blood sugar, postprandial blood sugar, and if warranted, a glucose tolerance test as well as a careful evaluation of diet to eliminate diabetes and/or high carbohydrate consumption as contributing factors. Older women with diabetes should be aware of increased risks of vaginitis. Coffee, tea, alcohol, and spices appear to be irritating to the bladder. If the woman is prone to cystitis, suggest she try eliminating these and drink lots of water or juice.

Women who are postmenopausal have special dietary needs to maintain health, supply energy requirements, and prevent problems. The amount of physical energy, use of drugs, weight, height, general build, and presence of chronic disease must all be considered in planning for adequate nutritional intake.[1]

Drugs

Use of antibiotics suppresses not only the offending organisms, but normal bowel and vaginal flora as well. Women on antibiotics for acne, as well as for infections, should be aware of the risk of monilia yeast infections. Eating lactobacillus yogurt or taking lactobacillus tablets seems to restore normal flora and prevent diarrhea, which often occurs as well when one is on antibiotics. This is especially important for older clients who may be debilitated and more susceptible to secondary infections. Because a woman is postmenopausal or posthysterectomy does not mean she is no longer susceptible to vaginal infections.

Intercourse

Pain is a fairly common problem encountered by sexually active women, but one that, barring anatomic anomaly or pathology, need not occur. It is usually related to infection or irritation in or around the vagina and may also be related to insufficient lubrication and/or insufficient foreplay. Treatment and prevention of recurrence of infection should eliminate pain from that cause. If lubrication is insufficient, extending foreplay and using a finger in foreplay to bring lubrication down from the upper portion of the vagina where it begins may help. Saliva or a water soluble gel may be used to supplement natural lubrication.

In women who are postmenopausal or who have had a hysterectomy and oophorectomy, vaginal atrophy may occur, diminishing output of lubrication due to decrease in estrogen. Time for lubrication to occur extends often to several minutes.[2(pp39-40)] Topical use of estrogen through vaginal creams or suppositories may help. These make the vaginal mucosa more lush and are also useful for treating irritation around the urinary meatus. Because topical estrogen products are absorbed, they should be used only when other interventions fail and then sparingly and with caution. These are absorbed directly into the blood, bypassing the liver. Thus, this may be a more risky means of administering estrogen than orally. The woman who is sexually active on a regular basis will probably incur far less atrophy of the vagina than the woman who has not been active for an extended period of time.

After menopause, loss of tissue elasticity, thinning and atrophy of the vaginal walls, and decrease in the size of the vaginal vault may contribute to discomfort during intercourse.[2(p39)] The uterus may not elevate as much as in younger women, so penile thrusting against the cervix may occur and be painful. The orgasmic phase may be shorter and uterine contractions more spastic and painful. Hot flushes, dizziness, headaches, and exhaustion may also occur. Vaginal, clitoral, bladder, labial, and urethral sensitivity are more common in women after menopause[2(pp40-41)] and demand sensitivity of the partner and good communication in order to assure a continuation of positive sexual experiences.

In the woman who has undergone a hysterectomy without oophorectomy, gradual decline in ovarian function and resultant symptoms occur. If the ovaries are removed, symptoms are immediate. Dyspareunia due to shortening of the vagina, and tender scar tissue is common until healing is complete.[2(p41)]

For the young woman whose body is anatomically immature, pain may be due to stretching of the hymenal ring or the vagina, penile pressure on the cervix during thrusting, inadequate lubrication, and lack of knowledge about sexual response and technique. The setting for a first sexual experience is extremely important. Guiding a woman in decision making about her sexual experiences can help her to feel more control over her own body and where and with whom sex occurs. Some women need support and reassurance that it is okay to say no and to reserve intercourse for a time and person with whom they feel comfortable in sharing intimacy. Pain, discomfort, and even tissue damage can occur when the woman is immature physically and not ready for intercourse emotionally and feels trapped or forced into an undesired encounter.

Pain may be related to the depth and angle of penetration. Counseling the woman as to different positions to alter penetration may relieve the discomfort. An understanding of the anatomy of both partners will help each to be more sensitive to the needs and comfort of the other.

It is always important to rule out pathology that may cause pain. Fibroids and other tumors, lesions, masses in the adnexa, and ovarian cysts all may be sensitive to pressure and touch. Anomalies in structure, cystoceles, cystitis, rectoceles, and prolapse of the uterus may cause pain with intercourse. Pelvic inflammatory disease and ectopic pregnancy may produce acute pain. Referral should be made whenever the cause is in question or cannot be found and suggestions for elimination of pain do not help.

Pelvic congestion and a feeling of heaviness are problems for women, most commonly for those who are not orgasmic. They are due to the vasocongestion that is part of sexual response and is relieved when orgasm occurs. Exploration of feelings about sex, arousal, and timing of intercourse will help to identify the cause—whether it be related to the complexity of feelings or to lack of adequate stimulation. Masturbation to orgasm may help the woman to recognize signs of arousal and identify her own responsiveness. It is important, however, to be aware of and respect cultural and religious taboos regarding masturbation. Communication of her needs to her partner is an essential part of a satisfying experience for both. Referral to a person whose specialty is sexual therapy or counseling may be considered for women open to such a suggestion.

Prevention of infection is paramount if sex is to be a comfortable and satisfying experience. Communication about exposure to infection is part of a trust relationship. So is compliance with treatment (such as use of a condom) to eliminate recurrence. Good hygiene is a key to prevention of infection. Urinating before and after intercourse will reduce trauma to the bladder and wash organisms out of the urethra. Clean hands and genitalia of both partners will aid in preventing infection and avoiding pain or irritation. If the woman is prone to develop cystitis, she should avoid stretching or traumatizing the urethra during intercourse. After a bout of cystitis, she should also avoid positions that will put excessive pressure on the bladder, irritating newly healed mucosa. Positions such as rear entry either prone or standing bent over and the woman sitting on top and leaning forward may be uncomfortable and cause trauma until healing is complete.

A partner with fungus on feet, inner thighs, groin, or buttocks can transfer this fungus to the partner, who may then develop a vaginal yeast infection. Sometimes it is necessary to query as to existence of such acute or chronic episodes of fungus in order to break the cycle of infections from one partner to another. Over-the-counter products are available to help eradicate and prevent recurrence of topical fungal infections.

Contraception

Part of primary prevention is teaching about contraceptive measures for those women desiring to prevent or postpone pregnancy. Contraceptive counseling requires adequate time, respect for the woman's (or couple's) right to make her own decision, and support during the decision-making process.

When working with young adolescent girls, be alert to the possibility of sexual activity. Clients who present for routine care and who give an extensive history of social activities or have evidence of a "hickey," those with repeated vague complaints or recurrent infections, and girls who might be runaways or emancipated minors are at particular risk for pregnancy.[3] Evaluating her knowledge of human sexuality, her own anatomy, and changes she is experiencing in puberty can help to bring discussion to the girl's own sexuality and sexual activity. Working through pregnancy risks with a sexually active adolescent can assist her in making a realistic decision about contraception.[3(p195)]

The means of contraception that may be offered to an adolescent are affected by developmental stage, both physical and social. Intrauterine devices for very young women are generally contraindicated due to high risk of infection and spontaneous rejection. Oral contraceptives given before establishment of regular ovulatory cycles may contribute to postpill amenorrhea and infertility due to anovulation. Also, beginning oral contraceptives in early teens may mean numerous years of use before a pregnancy is desired, and we know little about the long-term effects. Foam, condoms, and diaphragms require high user motivation and involvement.[3(p195)] Rhythm, particularly for a young woman who has not even established regular menstrual cycles, is highly unreliable and demands much self-control.

For older adolescents and young adults, the choices are a little easier and may be based on frequency of sexual activity, comfort with one's body, absence or presence of contraindications for a particular method, and user acceptance. Women contracepting between pregnancies may choose less reliable methods with fewer associated dangers or side effects, as a variation in spacing of children may be less important than risk taking. Women who have completed their families are faced with decisions for contracepting over their remaining years of fertility. Medical and gynecologic history may influence the choices, as well as age. Women over 35 years of age are generally advised to choose a method other than oral contraceptives. If another pregnancy would be disastrous either psychosocially or physically, the most effective methods or sterilization may be the only acceptable choices.

Women who are sexually active but have made the decision never to biologically parent are faced with the problem of long-term contraception or the choice of sterilization.

During the climacteric, women need accurate information about fertility in order to contracept safely until ovulation ceases completely. To ensure that an unwanted or unexpected pregnancy will not occur, one full year of uninterrupted amenorrhea must be experienced before discontinuing use of contraception. Although the last few cycles may be anovulatory, the risk of pregnancy is present until the year of amenorrhea occurs.

Because the average age of menarche lies somewhere between 10 to 14 (mean 12.8 years) and 50, a woman faces decisions concerning contraception for some 35 to 40 years of her life. With the declining size of families, women experience fewer pregnancies and, thus, more years of fertility and risk of unwanted pregnancy. Contraceptive counseling and teaching, therefore, form an important component of primary health care for women.

Abstinence

For most women, at one time or another during their 30-plus years of fertility, abstinence is the best choice. It is the most commonly used method of teenagers[4(p179)] and may be practiced for varying amounts of time by other women for many reasons. For teenagers, particularly, it may be the most appropriate choice when sexual activity is not desired, relationships are fragile and transient, and anatomical maturity has not yet been achieved. Teenagers often need support for the decision to abstain and reassurance that they are not abnormal. Sexual activity without intercourse—mutual masturbation, stroking, hugging, kissing, and other forms of touching and caressing—can provide means of sexual pleasure and expression without the risk of pregnancy and stresses of contraceptive decision making.[4(p180)]

Withdrawal

Withdrawal, probably the oldest and most widely used method, is not a means of avoiding pregnancy. Sperm are present in the lubricating secretions that accompany sexual arousal and precede orgasm and can be deposited even if ejaculation occurs outside the vagina. If ejaculation occurs on the labia or around the introitus, pregnancy risk is also great. Teenagers may find it difficult to control ejaculation in order to withdraw prior to its occurrence.

Rhythm and natural methods

Rhythm, or the calendar method, is based on computation of time of ovulation and, thus, the unsafe period. Because most women have cycles that are somewhat variable and subject to alterations by emotional and physical factors, the method is not very reliable. Additional practices can enhance the efficacy of rhythm.

A number of changes occur in a woman's body as a result of the pituitary ovarian feedback cycle. The woman can be taught to recognize these changes and their relationship to the fertile period of ovulation. During the first half of the cycle prior to ovulation, estrogen is the dominant hormone and causes the cervical mucus to be thin, slippery, and stringy and to form a ferning pattern visible with a microscope. After ovulation, the progesterone produced by the corpus luteum makes the cervical mucus thick, tacky, and opaque. As it is thermogenic, progesterone is also responsible for the rise in temperature, a shift that requires 24 hours or more after ovulation.[5(pp41-43)]

Women can use the basal body temperature as one index of fertility. The midcycle drop in temperature at ovulation followed by a sustained rise of about 0.4 F is due to progesterone production. By charting her cycles for at least six months, the woman can establish the earliest day of temperature rise and then subtract six days to establish the first day of fertility (see Figure 6.1).[5(pp44-45)]

Women can also observe the cervical mucus to determine peak of Spinnbarkheit when mucus is clear, slippery, lubricative, and stretchy and then resume vaginal intercourse four days after this peak (Billings method).[5(p45)]

In the press recently, reports of a method of birth control based on a series of physical measurements indicate an efficacy of 98 to 99%. Skeptics claim it works only with well-educated, highly motivated individuals with a high level of control. The method is advocated by the Couple-to-Couple League and is taught by trained lay couples. It is based on the rhythm or calendar method, calculating fertile periods, measuring the vaginal temperature, and observing cervical mucus changes.[6]

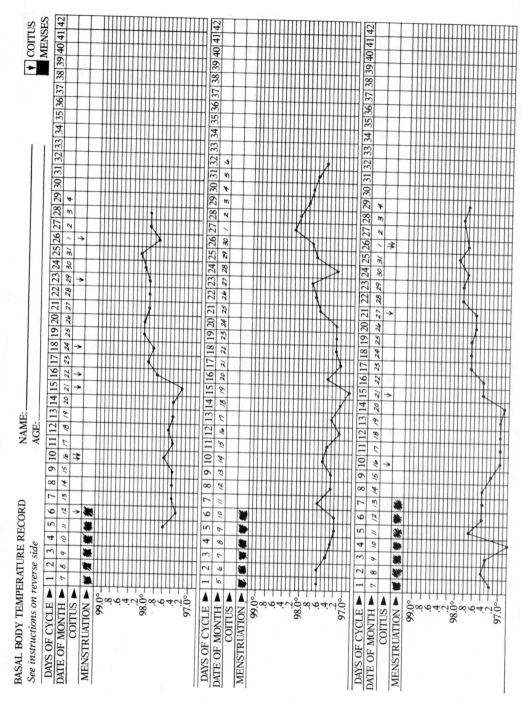

Figure 6.1 Basal Body Temperature Records

81

Other signs of ovulation can help the woman to determine the fertile period and when it is safe to resume intercourse. Some women experience Mittelschmerz, pain at the time of ovulation, probably due to follicular rupture and irritation of the peritoneum from the small amount of blood that may be extruded with the ovum. Women may notice preovulatory signs like fluid retention, alterations in appetite, odiferous or strange-smelling urine, diuresis with ovulation, distention of the lower abdomen, and change in libido. Most of these are very individual symptoms. As the woman becomes more aware of her body and understands the ovulatory and endometrial cycles, she may be able to detect more subtle, subjective signs of her fertility and correlate these with her temperature chart, the calendar, and cervical mucus. Sperm may live up to 72 hours after ejaculation and the ovum probably 12 to 24 hours, so the woman needs to calculate these figures into her fertile and safe periods.

Irregular cycles, transiency of relationships, and infrequent sexual activity make fertility awareness a method that is not very safe for most teenagers. It may be suggested as an alternative or backup to other methods. For the woman for whom this is the only acceptable method, counseling about taking basal body temperature, signs of ovulation, mucus changes, life span of sperm and the ovum, and calculation of unsafe periods during which she must abstain are all important.

Condoms and foam

Condoms and vaginal foam in combination are a fairly effective means of contraception. If sensitivity to rubber or to the spermicide in foam occurs, switching to condoms made of the cecum of lambs or to a different brand of foam may help. The active spermicidal ingredient is usually nonylphenoxypolyoxyethylene ethanol. Dissipation of foam produces vaginal discharge that some women find unpleasant. Foam is also available in suppository and effervesced forms. Spermicidal suppositories may either effervesce or melt by body heat and spread spermicide around the cervix. The package inserts often say 10 minutes are required for effectiveness, but 20 minutes may be more realistic for melting or effervescence to be completed and the cervix swathed in spermicide. These products seem to be less effective than more traditional foam and cause more irritation (see Figure 6.2).

The chief disadvantage of condoms and foam is that they must be inserted or applied at the time of sexual arousal. A full applicator of foam must be inserted deep into the vagina so it surrounds the cervix within half an hour before intercourse. Instruct the woman to shake the canister well, 15 to 20 times. The condom must be rolled on the erect

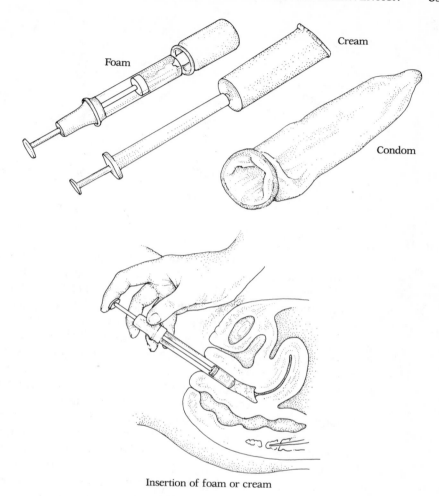

Foam

Cream

Condom

Insertion of foam or cream

Figure 6.2   Vaginal Contraceptive Foam or Cream and the Condom

penis, leaving a reservoir at the tip for the ejaculate. Saliva or lubricating jelly can be used on the condom if desired. Vaseline should not be used as it deteriorates rubber. Some condoms are ribbed, some lubricated, some colored, and some have a reservoir tip. After ejaculation, the penis should be carefully withdrawn, holding the condom so it does not slip off. Condoms should be used only once, but may be reused if carefully washed, tested for leaks and powdered with cornstarch.[7(p33)] Some men complain that condoms decrease pleasure.

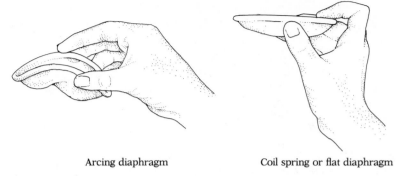

Arcing diaphragm   Coil spring or flat diaphragm

Figure 6.3   Two Types of Diaphragms

Diaphragms

Diaphragms are fitted individually. They usually range in size from 65 to 90 ml in diameter and come with flat, arcing, or coil springs (see Figure 6.3). Diaphragms smaller than 65 ml and larger than 90 ml are available but may have to be special-ordered. The arcing spring is the one most commonly used as it regains shape readily after insertion, which aids in proper placement. It has a firmer spring than the others and thus may be less comfortable. Contraindications to diaphragm use include sensitivity to rubber or spermicide, inability to fit properly, chronic constipation, anomalies of uterus, inadequate pubic arch, and unwillingness on the part of the woman to touch herself for insertion or removal.

A diaphragm must always be used with one to one and a half teaspoons of spermicidal jelly or cream, may be inserted four hours or fewer prior to intercourse without adding more spermicide to the outside of the diaphragm, and must be left in place at least six to eight hours after the last intercourse. For repeat intercourse or when more than four hours have elapsed since insertion, instruct the woman to add another teaspoon of jelly or cream to outside of diaphragm with an applicator or her fingers. Tell her not to douche while using a diaphragm. The diaphragm should be washed and dried thoroughly and may be dusted with cornstarch.

Fitting a diaphragm takes practice and someone to check the fit until the woman feels confident. Once the optimal size—snug without causing pain, discomfort, or pressure—is reached, the woman should be allowed to insert and remove it a couple of times and her technique checked before she is given a prescription. Also have her feel her cervix through the diaphragm so she can tell when the diaphragm is in place properly covering the cervix. If she has never used a diaphragm before, it may be desirable to have her return in a week to check the fit and review use. Choice of jelly or cream is a matter of personal preference. If sensitivity to one occurs, suggest trying the other or switching brands. Contraceptive foam should not be used and neither should vaseline, as they both will cause the rubber to deteriorate.

Most important to successful diaphragm use are selection of this method as appropriate for the woman, proper fitting, and adequate teaching. Good teaching requires time for feedback and for evaluation of effectiveness so that misinformation is not the end product (see Figures 6.4–6.6).[8,9(p24)]

With proper teaching, familiarity of the woman with her own anatomy, and time for her to practice insertion and removal, diaphragm failures are considerably lessened.[10] Teens and younger women not previously sexually active should be checked for diaphragm fit more frequently than once a year. The woman who has gained or lost more than 10 to 15 pounds, has had an abortion or a pregnancy, or is experiencing difficulty inserting or removing her diaphragm after the initial teaching should be seen to have the fit checked. Failures are most commonly related to improper fit, dislodgement due to vaginal wall expansion and coital position,[11] and inadequate teaching or understanding of use. Some protocols suggest use of condoms around the time of ovulation for extra protection (see Appendix).[12(p134)]

Oral contraceptives

There is a plethora of brands of oral contraceptives on the market. Each setting in which you practice will have certain preferred brands and protocols for choices. Each setting will have its own protocol for compliance with the FDA's ruling that women must give informed consent when prescribed any estrogen preparations. Some clinics require classes, use printed material, and have the client review and sign a consent form. A chart comparing types of hormones and dose is useful in making the initial choice and in evaluating problems (see Table 6.1).

Poor candidates for oral contraceptives are women with a history of elevated blood pressure, varicosities, diabetes, migraines, heart or vascular disease, hepatitis, jaundice, elevated cholesterol, breast or reproductive malignancy, sickle cell anemia, phlebitis, grand mal epilepsy, undiagnosed vaginal bleeding, severe varicosities, or evidence of liver damage. Those who are lactating or possibly pregnant, have irregular menses or fewer than ten periods a year, smoke, or are over 35 also seem to run greater risks. Women who are on another form of hormonal therapy, such as steroids, are usually not placed on oral contraceptives. A

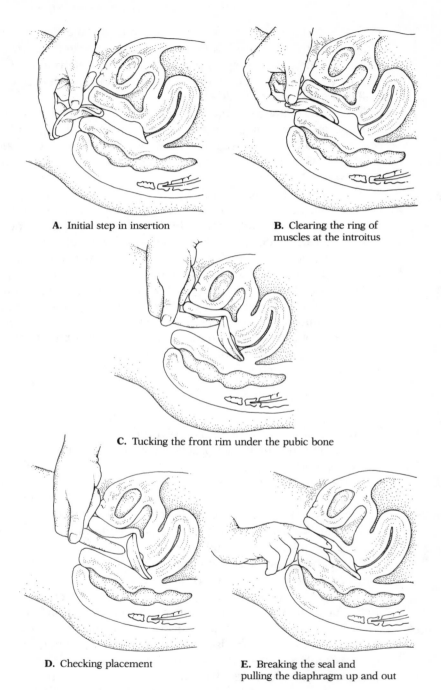

A. Initial step in insertion

B. Clearing the ring of
muscles at the introitus

C. Tucking the front rim under the pubic bone

D. Checking placement

E. Breaking the seal and
pulling the diaphragm up and out

Figure 6.4 . Inserting and Removing a Diaphragm

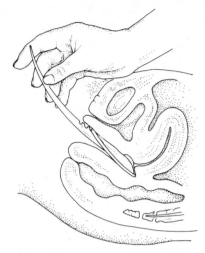

Figure 6.5   Inserting a Diaphragm Using an Introducer

careful history and physical examination are necessary before oral contraceptives are considered.

If by physical examination and history, the woman seems to be a likely candidate for oral contraceptives, a trial period of three months or so may be chosen. The low-dosage pills in use today are rapidly excreted, so it is important that the woman take the pill at the same time each day. If she misses taking a pill by more than six hours, back-up contraception for seven days may be recommended. If she misses a day, she should take the pill as soon as she remembers and is advised to use back-up contraception for the remainder of that pill cycle.

It is usual to begin the pill on the fifth day of the cycle or the Sunday after the onset of menses and take the 20 or 21 pills, stop for a week, and begin again. Some packets have seven inert or iron pills so that the woman always takes a pill.

Special consideration must be given in evaluating oral contraceptive use for a teenager who has not yet established regular ovulatory cycles or for a woman who gives a long-term history of irregular menses. There is concern that the pill may suppress the hypothalamus so ovulation will never occur. There is also concern that in young teens hormones will cause premature closure of the epiphyses. Others argue that pregnancy hormones would limit growth even more so.[12(p130)] Adolescents also need to know that there are many types of oral contraceptives, that they should not borrow from friends,[4(p182)] and that these do not work as "morning after pills."

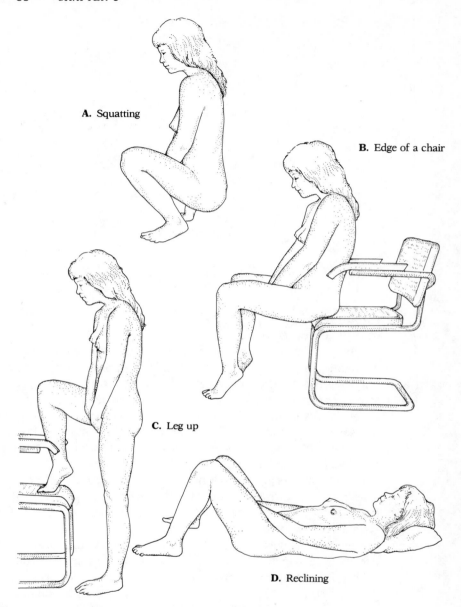

A. Squatting

B. Edge of a chair

C. Leg up

D. Reclining

Figure 6.6   Positions for Inserting a Diaphragm

TABLE 6.1 Oral Contraceptives: Formula and Dosage

| Brand Name | Progestogen Content in mg | | | | | Estrogen Content mcg | | | |
	Estrogenic effect 2.08 NORETHYNODREL Androgenic effect 0	Estrogenic effect 0.25 NORETHINDRONE Androgenic effect 1.6	Estrogenic effect 0.86 ETHYNODIOL DIACETATE Androgenic effect 1.0	Estrogenic effect 0.38 NORETHINDRONE ACETATE Androgenic effect 2.5	Estrogenic effect 0 NORGESTREL Androgenic effect 7.6	MESTRANOL	ETHINYL ESTRADIOL	# HORMONAL	# Other
Brevicon-21		0.5					35	21	
Brevicon-28		0.5					35	21	7 Inert
Demulen-21			1.0				50	21	
Demulen-28			1.0				50	21	7 Inert
Enovid 5	5.0					75		20	
Enovid E	2.5					100		21	
Loestrin 1/20				1.0			20	21	7 Iron
Loestrin 1.5/30				1.5			30	21	7 Iron
Lo/Ovral					0.3		30	21	
Lo/Ovral-28					0.3		30	21	7 Inert
Modicon-21		0.5					35	21	
Modicon-28		0.5					35	21	7 Inert
Norinyl 2 mg		2.0				100		20	
Norinyl 1+50/21		1.0				50		21	
Norinyl 1+50/28		1.0				50		21	7 Inert
Norinyl 1+80/21		1.0				80		21	
Norinyl 1+80/28		1.0				80		21	7 Inert
Norlestrin 2.5/50-21				2.5			50	21	
Norlestrin 2.5/50-FE				2.5			50	21	7 Iron
Norlestrin 1/50-21				1.0			50	21	
Norlestrin 1/50-28				1.0			50	21	7 Inert
Norlestrin 1/50-FE				1.0			50	21	7 Iron
Ortho-Novum 1/35/28		1.0					35		7 Inert
Ortho-Novum 1/35/21		1.0					35		
Ortho-Novum 2 mg		2.0				100		21	
Ortho-Novum 10 mg		10.0				60		20	
Ortho-Novum 1/50-21		1.0				50		21	
Ortho-Novum 1/50-28		1.0				50		21	7 Inert
Ortho-Novum 1/80-21		1.0				80		21	
Ortho-Novum 1/80-28		1.0				80		21	7 Inert
Ovcon-35		0.4					35	21	7 Inert
Ovcon-50		1.0					50	21	7 Inert
Ovral					0.5		50	21	
Ovral-28					0.5		50	21	7 Inert

TABLE 6.1 (*Continued*)

| | Progestogen Content in mg | | | | | Estrogen Content mcg | | | |
	Estrogenic effect 2.08 NORETHYNODREL Androgenic effect 0	Estrogenic effect 0.25 NORETHINDRONE Androgenic effect 1.6	Estrogenic effect 0.86 ETHYNODIOL DIACETATE Androgenic effect 1.0	Estrogenic effect 0.38 NORETHINDRONE ACETATE Androgenic effect 2.5	Estrogenic effect 0 NORGESTREL Androgenic effect 7.6	MESTRANOL	ETHINYL ESTRADIOL	# HORMONAL	# Other
Ovulen 20			1.0			100		20	
Ovulen 21			1.0			100		21	
Ovulen 28			1.0			100		21	7 Inert
Zorane 1/20				1.0			20	21	7 Inert
Zorane 1.5/30				1.5			30	21	7 Inert
Zorane 1/50				1.0			50	21	7 Inert
"MINI"									
Micronor		.35						35	
Nor-Q-D		.35						42	
Ovrette					.075			28	

Adapted from:
  Ericson A (ed): *Pharmacy Newsletter*. Boston, Boston Hospital for Women, 1977, vol 2.
  Gyn Family Planning Nurse Practitioners: *A Manual of Standard Practice Procedures and Policies*, Storrs, Conn, University of Connecticut Women's Health Clinic, 1980, p 6.
  Hatcher RA, et al: *Contraceptive Technology 1980–1981*, ed 10. New York, Irvington, 1980, pp 24–25, 27–28.

Danger signs the woman needs to know include loss or blurring of vision, spots before her eyes, numbness of face or body, chest pain, calf pain, severe headaches, increase in blood pressure, marked fluid retention or weight gain, severe mood changes or depression, and abdominal pain, especially in the area of the liver. Any of these should be reported at once and investigated.

Side effects such as midcycle spotting, skin rash, nausea, loss of hair, fatigue, headaches, change in libido, dyspareunia, fluid retention, weight gain, weight loss, amenorrhea, milk in breasts, chloasma, and vaginal discharge should be evaluated during the trial period and a switch in dosage made or the pill discontinued and an alternate method selected if necessary or desired. Some of these, of course, have other unrelated causes, which should be sought and treated. A summary of side effects is given in Table 6.2.

TABLE 6.2 Oral Contraceptives: Common Side Effects and Their Management

Side Effect	Possible/Probable Cause	Management
Nausea, abdominal pains	High-estrogen pill	Change to lower-estrogen pill; change type of estrogen
	Taking pills on empty stomach	Take with meal or snack
	G i virus or reaction to food	Rule out other causes and treat
Headaches	Estrogen	Low-estrogen pill
	Severe migraine (have before OC?)	Discontinue; MD consult
	Histamine reaction between pill packets	Higher-estrogen pill
	Occur before pill due to school or work pressure, tension, economic or social problems, lack of sleep	History to sort out cause
	Too much TV, poor light for TV or reading	Referral for eye check
	Premenstrual tension	
	Vision problems	Monitor B/P carefully
	Hypertension	Lower salt use
	Anemia	Check hematocrit
Weight gain	Increased appetite	Change to estrogen-dominant pill; low-androgen pill, low-estrogen pill
	Poor diet	Elicit diet history, diet counseling and teaching
	Hypertension and edema	Monitor, MD consult, may need to change method
	Emotional	Counseling
	Physical release from pregnancy	Observe for 3–6 months more
Weight loss	Poor appetite	Query cause
	No time to eat	Schedules, priorities, social
	Emotional or social	Counseling, referral as needed
	Medical problems, anemia, TB, hyperthyroid	Careful history and physical, MD referral
	With nausea or vomiting	Low estrogen with high progesterone, consider anorexia nervosa in young client
	Fear of OC effects	Explore comfort with method, fears
	Imagination	Compare weight records, history, progestin dominant pills
Fatigue	Anemia	Hematocrit, hemoglobin, diet history, teaching
	Infection	Careful history and physical, MD referral
	Overwork, lack of sleep, insomnia	Careful history, help set priorities
	Poor diet habits	Referral for counseling—social and academic as needed
Spotting, bleeding	Improper taking of pills: delay of more than 7 days between packs,	History of use—any missed, time of day, reassurance of normalcy

TABLE 6.2 (*Continued*)

Side Effect	Possible/Probable Cause	Management
	mix-up of 28-day packets, takes only before or after coitus, never stops taking OC with 20- or 21-day packet	when first on OC
	Vaginitis, cervical ectropion	Pelvic exam, smears, cultures as indicated; Pap smear yearly
	Gyn pathology—polyps, cysts, tumors, DES exposure	Check history of DES exposure
	OC	Early cycle (pill 1–14)—higher estrogen; late cycle (pill 15–21)—higher progesterone pill
Amenorrhea	Taking 20 or 21 pills without 1 week break	Check use of OC
	Pregnancy	Pregnancy test, pelvic exam
	Prolonged use of OC	Switch to higher estrogen for few months, another method for few months, endocrine work-up
Milk in breast	Pill use	
	Pregnancy	Pelvic exam, pregnancy test
	Sucking on breasts, foreplay, squeezing nipples, especially after pregnancy, abortion	Other forms of sexual stimulation until milk disappears
	Pituitary disorder	MD consult
	Use of other drugs: tranquilizers, heroin, morphine	Query as to drug use, MD consult
	Breast pathology	SBE, exam by practitioner, referral, mammogram as needed
Chloasma	Estrogen excess	Low-estrogen pill
	Pregnancy	Pregnancy test, pelvic exam
	Other pathology—endocrine, lupus	Careful history, physical, referral
Scant menses	Long use of OC, especially high-androgen	Estrogen-dominant pill, nonandrogen progestin
	Pregnancy	History of pill use, pregnancy test, pelvic exam
Skin rash	If related to starting OC, due to pill	MD consult, try another brand of OC
	Localized, unrelated to OC use	MD consult, rule out infection, communicable diseases, syphilis
Fluid retention	Renal, vascular, cardiac pathology	MD consult, careful history and physical
	Cyclical, pedal edema—OC	Low-estrogen, consider another method
Loss of hair	Hair products, curling irons, ironing hair, dyes, straighteners, wig use	Careful history

TABLE 6.2 (*Continued*)

Side Effect	Possible/Probable Cause	Management
	Postpartum	Assure patient, cycles of hair in different stages—temporary
	Progestin-dominant—androgenic OC	Change to estrogen-dominant
	Pathology—endocrine, malignancy	MD referral
Loss of libido	Excess progestin	Lower-progestin, estrogen-dominant
	Scant estrogen—premenopausal women	MD consult
	Marital, sexual, social problems	History, counseling referral
	No orgasm, relationship stressors	Knowledge of anatomy and physiology, sexual responsiveness, need for foreplay
Excessive bleeding	High-estrogen OC	Change to low-estrogen, high-progestin
	PID, vaginitis, myomata, pelvic pathology, DES exposure	Pap smear, smears and cultures, pregnancy test, history, pelvic exam, MD referral
Dyspareunia	Pelvic, vaginal, cervical pathology, PID, VD	Pelvic exam, MD referral
	Scant lubrication, irritations due to clothing, soaps, deodorants, douching	Education on sexual arousal, foreplay, avoidance of irritants
	Severe retroversion or retroflexion of uterus	Position for coitus
Vaginal discharge	High-estrogen pill	Switch to low-estrogen
	Vaginitis, irritants, cervicitis, PID, VD	Pelvic exam, smears, cultures, MD consult
Hirsutism	High-progestin, androgenic pill	Low-progestin, nonandrogenic, estrogen-dominated
	Endocrine causes, Stein-Leventhal	History, physical, MD consult
Oily scalp, skin, acne	Androgenic, high-progestin	Low-progestin, nonandrogenic, estrogen-dominated
	Hygiene	Health teaching
Depression, labile moods	High-estrogen, high-progestin	Low-estrogen, low-progestin, may need to discontinue OC
	Social problems, school, peers, marriage, job	History, counseling, referral

*Adapted from:
Gyn Family Planning Nurse Practitioners: *A Manual of Standard Practice Procedures and Policies*, Storrs, Conn, University of Connecticut Women's Health Clinic, 1980, pp 9–14.
Hatcher RA, et al: *Contraceptive Technology, 1980–1981*, ed 10. New York, Irvington, 1980, pp 29–30.
Shapiro HI: *The Birth Control Book*. New York, Avon, 1978, pp 25–27.

Intrauterine devices

   Intrauterine devices are available in a number of sizes and types (see Figure 6.7). They may be made of inert plastic, wound with copper wire, or impregnated with progesterone. They are contraindicated in pregnancy or suspicion thereof, endometrial carcinoma, myomata, pelvic infection, septic abortion, ectopic pregnancy, endometritis, and uterine abnormalities. Consultation and careful evaluation are necessary for women with severe menorrhagia and dysmenorrhea, history of endocarditis or rheumatic heart disease, sickle cell disease, severe anemia,

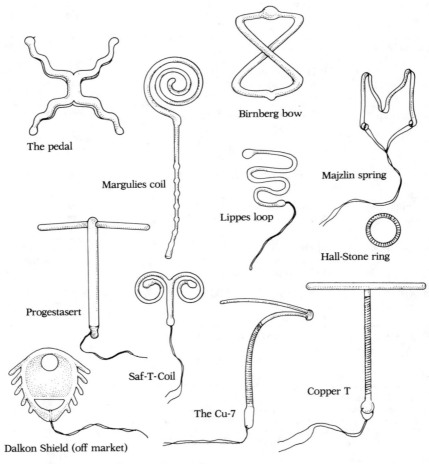

The pedal

Margulies coil

Birnberg bow

Lippes loop

Majzlin spring

Hall-Stone ring

Progestasert

Saf-T-Coil

The Cu-7

Copper T

Dalkon Shield (off market)

Figure 6.7 Types of Intrauterine Devices

gonorrhea in the past six months, Pap smear of Class III or greater, and for any woman on anticoagulents, with bleeding disorders, or with bleeding of unknown origin. A uterus of less than six centimeters depth is too small. Marked anteflexion or retroflexion increases danger of perforation on insertion.

Intrauterine devices are more likely to be retained in women who are parous. The smallest IUDs, copper and progesterone-impregnated, are best for adolescents. Complete assessment should be done prior to any decision to insert an IUD and careful explanation of dangers should be given. Insertion is usually done during menses to rule out pregnancy. The cervix is slightly dilated to facilitate insertion as well.

Dangers to report include pregnancy, prolonged or midcycle bleeding, severe cramps, signs of pelvic infection, amenorrhea, and inability to locate strings. After insertion, it is customary to instruct the woman to use an alternate method of birth control for the first four to eight weeks, the time when most spontaneous expulsions occur. To avoid infection of the uterus, for the first week nothing (including tampons, fingers, penis) should be inserted in the vagina. The woman should be shown how to check for strings, what they feel like, and when to check (usually after each menses). Many clinics ask the woman to return for a checkup 6 to 12 weeks after insertion, and then yearly for a Pap smear unless problems occur. Progesterone-impregnated IUDs must be changed yearly (as progesterone is used up), copper-wound every three years (as copper is dissipated), and some may be left in place for several years.[9(pp16-17),13] Common problems and management are cited in Table 6.3.

Cervical caps

Cervical caps, which are widely used in Europe, are still being investigated by the FDA (see Figures 6.8 and 6.9). The cervical cap covers the cervix and, in contrast to the diaphragm, is closely fitted and stays in place by suction. Recent research is producing custom-fitted caps. Work is progressing on a cap with a one-way valve so removal for menses will not be necessary.[14] Caps may be used with a small amount of spermicide and may be left in place for several days. Some practitioners advise women to remove them at least once every 24 hours to allow cervical mucus to be discharged. Queries as to long-term effects on cervical tissue remain unanswered. Present models are made of metal, hard plastic, or hard rubber. The cap is being widely dispensed through research projects on its use.[15] The cap, if it wins FDA approval, offers one more alternative to women.

TABLE 6.3 Common Problems with IUDs and Their Management

Side Effect/Problem	Possible/Probable Cause	Management
Cramps, spotting	Effects of insertion, sign of expulsion	Bimanual, speculum exam, history; if no pathology, wait; analgesics for cramps
	Infection	Pelvic exam, MD consult, remove IUD
Bleeding—prolonged, between menses	IUD expelled, dislodged	Pelvic exam, check length of strings; IUD in os—remove
	Incomplete abortion	History of delayed menses, bimanual exam, pregnancy test; MD consult
	PID	Cultures, exam; positive Chandelier's sign, MD consult, remove IUD
	Ectropion	Evaluate friability; Pap smear; MD consult
	Prolonged use	Removal, alternative method
	Gyn pathology	Evaluation, MD consult
Lower abdominal pain	Pelvic infection, pelvic pathology	History, exam, lab studies
	Gonorrhea	MD consult
	Cystitis	History, urine specimen
	Constipation	Diet history, bowel habits, teaching
	Appendicitis	Palpate, history, MD consult
	Ectopic pregnancy	Amenorrhea, scanty menses, adnexa tender, pregnancy test, MD referral
Lower back pain	Urinary	History, urine specimen
	Retroversion of uterus	Knee chest, change position of coitus
	Menstrual	Analgesics, remove IUD, prostaglandin inhibitors
	Orthopedic injury	History—injury, trauma, MD referral
	Gonorrhea	History, pelvic exam, cultures
Excessive menses	Presence of IUD	History of problem, history of bleeding—amount, clots, cramps, pelvic exam—rule out pathology, remove IUD
	Overlay of emotions, hormones	Reassurance, reevaluation
	Pelvic pathology: myomata, tumor, polyps, PID, vaginitis, endometriosis	Exam, MD consult
Delayed or scanty menses	Pregnancy	History, pregnancy test, pelvic exam, IUD in place?
	Postpartum amenorrhea, lactation amenorrhea	History, exam

TABLE 6.3 (*Continued*)

Side Effect/Problem	Possible/Probable Cause	Management
	Menopause	Age, other symptoms
	Endocrine	History, exam, MD referral, steroid therapy
	Drug reaction	Drug history, use of OC, pregnancy test
Vaginal discharge	Vaginitis, irritation	Type, amount, duration; symptoms; smears, cultures, pelvic exam
	Endometritis	Tenderness, positive Chandelier's, cultures, history, remove IUD
	Presence of IUD	Careful history, rule outs
Weight gain or loss	Change from OC	History, appetite, diet
	Change in diet, too much food, too busy	Careful diet history, counseling, MD referral
	Emotional stress	Counseling, MD referral
	Pathology	History, physical exam, MD referral
Dyspareunia	Device expelled or dislodged in os	Pelvic exam, presence of IUD, strings—length
	Vaginitis	History, exam
	Pelvic pathology	Exam, history
	Severe retroversion or retroflexion of uterus	Exam, knee-chest daily, alter coital position
	Marital or sexual problems	History, possible causes, MD referral, counseling, sexual techniques, lubrication, foreplay
	Cervical disease, ectropion, polyps, prolapse	Exam, MD referral
	Disease in pelvic organs	Referral to rule out bowel, bladder pathology
Can't feel strings	Improper instruction, afraid to touch self	Reassurance, teaching
	Expulsion	Speculum exam for presence, flat plate of abdomen if no strings and not detected in vagina, os; rule out pregnancy

Adapted from:
Gyn Family Planning Nurse Practitioners: *A Manual of Standard Practice Procedures and Policies.* Storrs, Conn, University of Connecticut Women's Health Clinic, 1980, pp 18–23.
Hatcher RA, et al: *Contraceptive Technology 1980–1981*, New York, Irvington, 1980, pp 65–75.
Huxall LK: Update on IUDs. *The American Journal of Maternal Child Nursing* 5: 186–190, 1980.

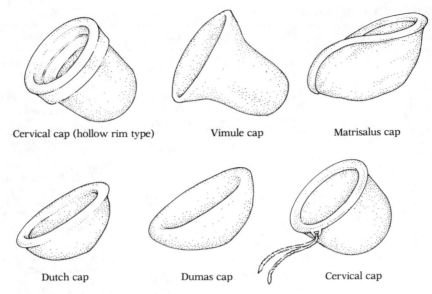

Cervical cap (hollow rim type)   Vimule cap   Matrisalus cap

Dutch cap   Dumas cap   Cervical cap

Figure 6.8   Types of Cervical Caps

Summary

It is important to ascertain whether or not a woman who comes for care is using or wishes to use contraception and to query her as to any problems or symptoms if she is contracepting. The woman needs to know, too, that loss of fertility after menopause or hysterectomy does not mean an end to sexuality. Freedom from fear of pregnancy may, in fact, enhance her feelings toward sex. Women may need support and help in exploring their sexuality at all ages and reassurance that sensuous and sexual feelings are not wrong at any time in the life span.[2]

SELF-CHECK

1. What would your approach be for the client in Chapter 1? Chapter 4?
2. What teaching would your plan include for each?
3. What differences might you anticipate for each of these clients due to age or other factors in relation to self-care practices, clothing, diet, and sexual activity?
4. Would your approach for these clients differ? If so, how? If not, why not?

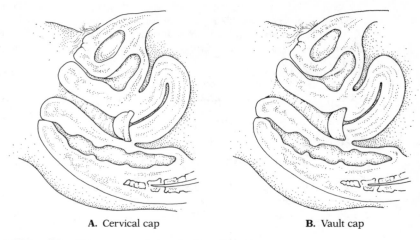

A. Cervical cap   B. Vault cap

Figure 6.9   Placement of Cervical and Vault Caps

References

1. Henley EC, Martin JB: Nutrition: a holistic approach for the older woman. *Issues in Health Care of Women* **1:** 15–36, 1978.
2. McKenzie CAM: Sexuality and the menopausal woman. *Issues in Health Care of Women* **1:** 39–44, 1978.
3. Peach EH: Counseling sexually active very young adolescent girls. *The American Journal of Maternal Child Nursing* **5:** 191–192, 1980.
4. Hatcher RA, et al: *Contraceptive Technology, 1980–1981*, ed 10. New York, Irvington, 1980.
5. Magenheimer EA: An alternative contraceptive method: fertility awareness. *Issues in Health Care of Women* **1:** 41–45, 1979.
6. Seymour G: 98% success claimed for birth control system. *The Hartford Courant* **163:** A30, 1980.
7. Wirth V: Condoms and foam: traditional forms of contraception still going strong. *Issues in Health Care of Women* **1:** 31–36, 1979.
8. Bradbury BA: Preventing the "diaphragm-baby syndrome": a matter of technique, teaching, and time. *Journal of Obstetric, Gynecologic and Neonatal Nursing* **4:** 25–32, 1974.
9. Gyn Family Planning Nurse Practitioners: *A Manual of Standard Practice Procedures and Policies.* Storrs, Conn, University of Connecticut Women's Health Clinic, 1980.
10. Lane ME, Arceo R, Sobrero AJ: Successful use of the diaphragm and jelly by a young population: report of a clinical study. *Family Planning Perspectives* **8:** 81–86, 1976.
11. Gorline LL: Teaching successful use of the diaphragm. *American Journal of Nursing* **79:** 1733, 1979.

12. Taylor D: Contraceptive counseling and care, in Mercer RT: *Perspectives on Adolescent Health Care.* Philadelphia, Lippincott, 1979.
13. Martin L: Gynecological problems, in Bullough B (ed): *The Management of Common Human Miseries.* New York, Springer Publishing, 1979, pp 106–107.
14. Willis M: Cervical caps: old and yet too new. *Science News* **116:** 431, 442, 1979.
15. Littman KJ: Contraception: the cervical cap. *Ms* **9:** 91–97, 1980.

For Further Reading

Boston Hospital for Women: The Oral Contraceptive Jungle. *Pharmacy Newsletter* 2, 1977.

Canavan, PA, Lewis, CA: The cervical cap: an alternative contraceptive. *Journal of Obstetric, Gynecologic and Neonatal Nursing* 10: 271–273, 1981.

Cooke CW, Dworkin S: *The Ms. Guide to a Woman's Health.* New York, Anchor Books, 1979.

Demarest RJ, Sciarra JJ: *Conception Birth Contraception.* New York, Hodder and Stoughton, 1969.

Hawkins JW, Higgins LP: *Maternity and Gynecological Nursing: Women's Health Care.* Philadelphia, Lippincott, 1981.

Hubbard CW: *Family Planning Education,* ed 2. St. Louis, CV Mosby, 1977.

Jones C: The first gynecological examination: establishing a partnership in health care. *Issues in Health Care of Women* 1: 3, 1979.

Shapiro HI: *The Birth Control Book.* New York, Avon, 1978.

Speroff L, Glass RH, Kase NG: *Clinical Gynecologic Endocrinology and Infertility,* ed 2. Chapter 11, Baltimore, Williams & Wilkins, 1978.

Zurek JG: *Looking Good Feeling Great.* Lombard, Ill, Joanne G Zurek, Publisher, 1978.

CHAPTER **7**

Breasts

At the end of Chapter 7, you will be able to:

1. synthesize knowledge of anatomy with information about breast examination
2. analyze the steps of breast examination
3. formulate a plan for breast examination of a client and incorporate teaching her the self-breast exam
4. describe common findings and deviations from normal

History Taking: Risk Factors

A family history of breast cancer—especially in mother, sister, maternal grandmother, or maternal aunt—increases risk of breast cancer in a woman. Women who have had no children or were primigravidas over age 30 are also at increased risk. Early menarche or late menopause are associated with a higher incidence of breast cancer. After age 40, risk increases significantly as it does for women who have had cancer of the reproductive organs or benign breast disorders.

Breast cancer is more common in White, Jewish, North American, and European women than it is in Black, African, non-Jewish, and Japanese women. Exposure to radiation for tuberculosis, treatment of postpartum mastitis, and chest irradiation in childhood for gynecomastia or hemangioma increase risk.[1]

The Examination

The woman should be seated and preferably stripped to the waist for the exam. In making this request, consider the woman's feelings about the examination. If she is uncomfortable being examined, utilize her clothing and/or a drape to cover her as much as possible during the procedure. It is her right to refuse the examination altogether so her consent and cooperation are essential before you begin.

Observe symmetry, color of areola, contours, and size of breasts. It is not uncommon for women to have one breast that appears slightly larger than the other. Color of skin, texture, and venous patterns should be the same for both breasts. Note any irregularities, masses, lumps, dimpling, or any orange peel-like appearance to the skin. Ask the woman if she has observed any changes. Observe any hair around the areola and the amount. Her nipples should be the same color, point in the same direction, and have no observable rashes or discharge. Nipples may be dimpled or inverted. If so, ascertain whether this is a change.

Have the woman raise her arms above her head and observe breasts for masses, lesions, ulcerations, dimpling, variations in appearance of skin, rashes, and contour. Ask her to place her hands on her hips and flex her chest muscles and again observe carefully. If breasts are large and pendulous, ask the woman to lean forward supported by a chair or by you, so you can assess her entire breasts.

With the woman in a dorsal recumbent position, place a small pillow or folded towel under the shoulder of the side to be examined. Ask the woman to raise her arm on that side and place her hand behind her head. This is the same position she can assume for self-breast examination while seated, lying down, or in the shower or tub.

Plan the examination so you always begin at the same place on the breast, moving in a clockwise fashion until you return to the area where you began. Because most tumors occur in the thickest area, the upper outer quadrant, many examiners choose to begin there. Using the pads of your middle three fingers in a rolling or circular motion, palpate the breast from periphery to nipple, following a pattern like the spokes of a wheel or concentric circles, moving clockwise until you have examined the entire breast (see Figure 7.1). Note the texture of tissue, nodules, any irregularities or granular sensation. It is common for women to experience tenderness, enlargement, and a feeling of fullness prior to onset of menses.

If you detect an irregularity, check the other breast. If you can feel the same structure in the same place in the other breast, it is probably normal, but worthy of observation through self-breast examination. Women with large breasts often have what feels like a distinctive ridge of tissue at the lower margin of each breast. In very thin women, ribs may be prominent and may feel like ridges or masses, especially in the lower quadrants.

Any nodules should be assessed for regularity, mobility, texture, size, location, sensitivity to touch, existence bilaterally, and whether they have discrete borders or blend into other tissues.

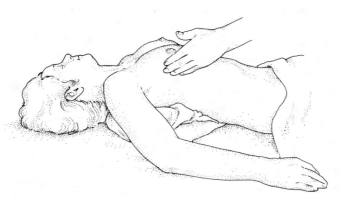

Figure 7.1   Palpation of Breast

Squeeze each nipple to express any discharge and check nipples for cracks, scaling, ulcerations, texture, integrity of tissue, color, and for any palpable lesions in areola or underneath. Palpate axillary nodes and note any enlargement or tenderness. Axillary nodes represent the usual first site of extension for breast tumors.[2,3]

Findings

Breasts should be relatively symmetrical, smooth, and without observable dimples, irregularities, or variations in skin color except for the areola. The nipples are normally everted and erectile (though some variations occur) and without discharge except during pregnancy and lactation. Axillary nodes, particularly the central ones, may be palpable but should not be enlarged or tender.

Common aberrations include long-standing inversion on one or both nipples, cyclical changes such as enlargement and tenderness, and enlarged milk glands or ducts. The latter are often granular in texture and are, by history, usually cyclical in occurrence and relatively symmetrical in both breasts. Women on oral contraceptives may experience enlargement and/or tenderness. They may also experience remission of symptoms of chronic cystic disease.

Dimpling, retraction, ulceration, inversion or deviation of a nipple, pig skin or orange peel texture of skin, alterations in contours, bloody nipple discharge, firm or hard nontender nodules are strongly suspicious of carcinoma. Any of these, occurring alone or together with other symptoms, is sufficient cause to warrant further evaluation.

Venous prominence and enlargement of breasts is often an early sign of pregnancy. Colostrum may be expressed at any time during pregnancy. Rarely, discharge may occur with use of oral contraceptives but it should always be investigated. Some drugs also cause discharge.[1(p207)]

Enlargement, inflammation, and infection of the hair follicles around the areola may occur spontaneously or in response to trauma such as attempts to remove unwanted hair. The cause for symptoms needs to be carefully assessed.

Some women have one or more additional breasts or nipples called supernumeraries. They occur along the nipple line from axilla to groin.

Chronic cystic disease, sometimes transitory with menstrual cycles, is manifested as one or more round, firm, well-defined mobile tender lesions. These may occur in clusters. Regression is usual postmenopausal and sometimes with use of oral contraceptives.

An adenofibroma is a benign lesion that usually presents as a firm, mobile, nontender round mass.

It is important to have any lesions you may find evaluated as differential diagnosis is very difficult. Any lesion should be treated as abnormal unless it is obvious by history, evaluation of the other breast, and/or timing of menses that it is a normal characteristic of that woman's breast.

Enlarged or tender axillary nodes should be evaluated as to possible causes. Reactions to deodorants or soaps, infection, or insult such as nicks when shaving may account for changes in nodes. If cause and effect seem certain, reevaluate once the proposed cause has been resolved or removed (for example, discontinue deodorant or allow the cut to heal). If nodes are enlarged or tender and no cause is detectable, refer the woman for further evaluation.

It is most important that you learn to recognize what is normal and to differentiate any deviations, assess as to any obvious possible causes, and refer for uncertainties or unknowns.

Plan and Interventions

Self-breast examination is an important part of taking responsibility for one's own health maintenance. Most breast tumors, about 90%, are first detected by women themselves. Although we cannot yet claim success in the battle against breast cancer, significant progress is being made. Many of its victims are now living long, productive lives.

If the woman you are caring for reports that she does self-breast examination, review with her the timing and techniques. You might ask her at what time of month she does the exam and to demonstrate for you the method she uses. If she has never done an exam before, assess her willingness to learn and her comfort in touching herself. Sometimes women who are very uneasy about touching themselves will allow their partners to do the exam.

For the observation phase of the exam, the woman should sit or stand in front of a mirror so that she can see her entire breasts. To palpate, she can sit with her arm elevated and hand behind her head, stand in the shower, or lie down with a small pillow or folded towel under her shoulder (see Figure 7.2). Teach her what to observe for and how to palpate, demonstrating and having her feed back information and return the demonstration. It is important to convey not only what and how but also why.

Timing of the examination is important. For the menstruating woman, the optimal time is around the fifth day of the cycle when hormone levels and influences are lowest. The woman who is taking oral contraceptives can do the self-breast exam on the fifth day (counting the day she begins to bleed as day one) or when she begins a new packet of pills.

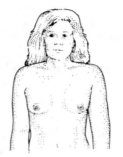

A. Stand with arms down.

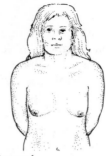

B. Lean forward.

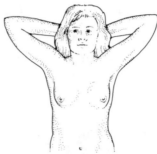

C. Raise arms overhead and press hands behind your head.

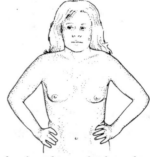

D. Place hands on hips and tighten chest and arm muscles by pressing firmly inward.

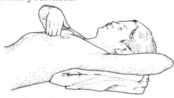

E. Lie with a pillow or folded towel under your left shoulder. Place your left arm above your head. With your right hand, feel the inner half of your left breast from top to bottom and from nipple to breastbone.

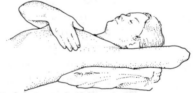

F. Feel the outer half from bottom to top and from the nipple to the side of the chest.

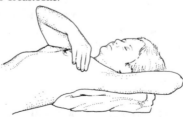

G. Pay special attention to the area between the breast and armpit itself.

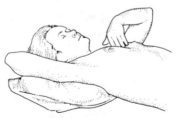

H. Now, place the pillow or towel under your right shoulder. Repeat this same process for your right breast using the fingers of your left hand to feel.

Figure 7.2   Self-Breast Examination

106

Postmenopausal women should choose a time of month and consistently check breasts at that time to minimize influences of any cyclical changes.

During pregnancy, breast changes are significant and breast examination is fraught with exceptions due to growth and development of milk glands and ducts and possible presence of colostrum. When women are doing breast exams, they need information about expected normal changes and some help in evaluating change during visits for prenatal care. Breast enlargement and tenderness may make self-examination difficult and painful.

Pamphlets available from the National Cancer Institute and the American Cancer Society can be used to supplement and reinforce verbal instructions and demonstrations.[4,5] These should not be a substitute for teaching, however, since those women who examine their breasts regularly tend to be those who were taught by a health worker. We as nurses in primary care can be understanding teachers in helping women to overcome their indifference and/or aversion to doing self-breast examination regularly as part of their own health care.

SELF-CHECK

1. How would you approach breast examination for each of the clients presented in Chapters 1–4?
2. What differences would you take into account?
3. Are these women at equal risk? If not, what factors would you evaluate as placing each woman at risk?
4. Outline a teaching plan for each of these clients.

References

1. Green TH Jr: *Gynecology—Essentials of Clinical Practice*, ed 3. Boston, Little, Brown, 1977.
2. Strax P: Screening for breast cancer. *Clinical Obstetrics and Gynecology* **20:** 797, 1977.
3. Bates B: *A Guide to Physical Assessment*, ed 2. Philadelphia, Lippincott, 1979.
4. *Breast Exams—What You Should Know.* Bethesda, Md, US Dept of Health, Education and Welfare, Public Health Service, National Cancer Institute, 1980.
5. *How to Examine Your Breasts.* American Cancer Society, 1975.

For Further Reading

Breast Cancer Annotated Bibliography of Public, Patient, and Professional Information and Educational Materials. Bethesda, Md, US Dept of Health,

Education and Welfare, Public Health Service, National Institutes of Health, 1979.

The Breast Cancer Digest. A Guide to Medical Care, Emotional Support, Educational Programs and Resources. Bethesda, Md, US Dept of Health, Education and Welfare, Public Health Service, National Institutes of Health, 1979.

Haagenen CD: *Diseases of the Breast*, ed 2. Philadelphia, Saunders, 1971.

Townsend CM: Breast lumps, *Clinical Symposia*, vol 32. Summit, NJ, CIBA, 1980.

CHAPTER *8*

Health Care of Women

Women are no longer a passive, docile, and compliant group of health-care recipients. The rebirth of the spirit of feminism, the growth of the consumer movement, and an increased awareness of ethical issues by professionals and the public have served to notify health care providers that women clients will no longer blindly obey all directives.

Nurses, most of whom are women, must be informed about the health-care activities of their own sex. In order that deeper schisms not develop between consumers and providers of health care, nurses need to keep open minds and open channels of communication with lay groups.

The Feminist Movement

Perhaps one of the most important outcomes of modern feminism is women's determination to learn about and care for their own bodies. That underlying feeling of shame associated with "women's problems" has given way to a feeling of pride in physical womanhood.

The self-help/self-health movement came about as a response by women to what was perceived as inadequate, often sexist, and inhumane care at the hands of health professionals. The early 1970s gave birth to many groups of women whose purposes were to discuss problems encountered within the traditional medical care system, to share experiences, and to seek out information. One group, the Boston Women's Health Book Collective, wrote a highly successful book, *Our Bodies, Ourselves.*[1] The overwhelming acceptance of and interest in this book is an indication of the depth of the need for such knowledge.

Self-help has come to mean women's active participation in their own health care. It assumes the individual's right to make decisions regarding her body and encompasses a holistic approach to care. This self-help movement eliminates the status differences between providers and consumers. The "patient" role disappears and is replaced with a participant role. The movement encourages women's concern for other women, a concern that mandates safe equipment and practices as well as competent professional back-up.

Unlike men's genitals, which can be seen and touched by their owners at will, women's reproductive organs remain hidden and mysterious. Women in self-help groups have begun to decrease the enigmas of their own bodies. One way this has been done is through the use of vaginal speculums enabling women to visualize their own and others' cervixes. Because the cervix is an important barometer of reproductive health, the trained eye can perceive a great deal by its visualization. Women who mastered the technique became familiar with their own cervixes and, over a period of time, learned to interpret the meaning of changes they observed. They found they could discern the difference between a normal cervix and an abnormal one. They were able to associate certain color and mucus changes with the menstrual cycle. They could spot infection early and begin treatment promptly.

These groups of health professionals are interested in improving health care and consider prevention of illness a high priority. As women begin to understand the workings of their bodies, they become better equipped to care for themselves. They begin to see the relationship between good health habits and health. For example, the effects of good dietary and sleep patterns may be reflected in reproductive health.

Some self-help groups teach the technique of menstrual extraction, which is a powerful method of exercising control over one's body. With a small plastic cannula and a suction device such as a syringe, the monthly flow can be aspirated in about five minutes on the first day of the period. Even though most users of menstrual extraction do not advocate the procedure as a method of birth control or abortion, it is sometimes used for those purposes.

The self-help movement logically led to the development of self-help or women-run clinics. These operations often operate on a shoestring. Women who work in these clinics may receive very little financial remuneration, but the money is divided equally among all workers as are the tasks. The care providers do not erect barriers between themselves and their clients. The clinics give more than lip service to the belief that health care should include education. Patients are present when their own pregnancy tests are done. The care providers often demonstrate breast self-examination on themselves. Many self-help clinics offer abortion services, counseling, and contraception information. People from the clinics are often willing to present programs for lay or professional audiences.

Another aspect of women's health care that the feminist movement has helped to examine has to do with sexual preference. The client who needs health care may be heterosexual, bisexual, lesbian, celibate, and/or autoerotic. The nurse needs to examine her own feelings and attitudes about sexual beliefs and practices that differ from her own. The heterosexual nurse, for example, may learn from her lesbian clients what their special health care needs are.

As greater numbers of nurses become aware of women's special health needs and the barriers that often prevent their recognition, high-quality care for all women may become a reality.

Consumerism

The consumer movement has resulted in a public that is better-informed about the goods and services it purchases. Quality health care at reasonable cost is among those services which knowledgeable consumers are demanding. The Health Planning and Resources Development Act of 1974 includes stipulations that consumers must sit on boards of the health systems agencies. Because women make more visits to physicians than men, it is often women who become involved in neighborhood health centers. Many women's organizations have been actively involved in leafleting, speaking, educating, and supporting women's right of control over their bodies. Many others belong to groups that condemn abortion as evil. These activities indicate that a great number of women are becoming politicized and are willing to fight for what they believe is right.

In the course of their daily practices, nurses will meet women who have a variety of values about health care and their own bodies. These values reflect their cultures, religious beliefs, and other traditions. The nurse will find that her teaching and counseling will be more effective if she strives to understand her client's culture. For example, if a nurse decides that a diaphragm would be the ideal form of contraception for a particular client without realizing that her client believes that "touching herself" is dirty, the nurse's teaching will not be heard. A careful assessment includes listening to the client's request for care and meeting the client's expectations within the boundaries of professional standards of care.

The nurse working with gynecology patients may appear to be involved in a narrow field. The knowledgeable nurse, however, is not only secure in administering physical care but has in-depth knowledge of growth and development. Such a nurse can just as easily minister to a budding woman of 15 who fears she has a venereal infection as to a mature postmenopausal women who is suffering from dyspareunia. Women of all ages require sensitive, respectful, and safe health care.

Increased Interest in Ethical Issues

The burst of scientific knowledge and proliferation of technology in the second half of this century have led to some marvelous life-saving and life-prolonging devices. With these advances have come questions about life-and-death issues that eventually, in some way, touch each one of us. Out of concern for self-determination and fear that inhumanity goes hand in hand with machinery, health care workers, philosophers, and others began to seek out answers.

Merely a few years ago, nurses were instructed to keep information away from their clients. In contrast, the modern nurse will be on shaky ground both ethically and legally if she or he does not allow the client to participate in decisions about her care. Because one area of concern involved research and experimentation, the federal government established guidelines for informed consent. The use of these guidelines is becoming standard practice in everyday matters between health-care providers and receivers. Essentially the guidelines are:

- the client must be given an explanation of the procedures including discomforts, risks, and benefits
- the client must be told if the procedure is experimental
- alternative procedures must be described with their risks and benefits
- an offer must be made to answer the client's questions
- the client must be told that consent may be withdrawn at any time.

Clients need to be involved in making decisions about their own bodies. In order to do that, they need enough information with which to make informed decisions. If a client makes a decision that is contrary to the nurse's value system, the client still has the right to receive safe health care. If the client decides to have an abortion and that decision is abhorrent to her nurse, what responsibility does that nurse have? The Nurse's Association of the American College of Obstetricians and Gynecologists published a statement on abortion and sterilization that reads in part: "Nurses have the right to refuse to assist in the performance of abortions and/or sterilization procedures in keeping with their moral, ethical, and/or religious beliefs, except in an emergency when a patient's life is clearly endangered in which case the questioned moral issue should be disregarded."[4(p61)]

Legal Issues

Every nurse must be cognizant of those legal constraints and protections which influence his or her practice. Statutory law, which is the result of legislation, forms the basis of the nurse practice acts of every state. The practice acts may be written in a general way or may be quite specific. However, nearly all states have dealt with the expanded role of the nurse. The method used varies with the individual state. Some states have simply left the laws unchanged but are interpreting them more liberally; others have amended the statutes by authorizing expanded practice; the remainder have allowed the professional nurse-licensing boards to issue rules and regulations. The nurse who is practicing in an expanded role must be knowledgeable about the nurse practice acts in his or her state.

The other form of the law, derived from previous court cases, is called common law or common law of torts. Issues that involve malpractice are disputed under tort law.

Laws that have a less direct impact on nursing practice may nonetheless influence to a great extent the practice of the profession. For example, laws governing third-party payments for services have traditionally excluded nurses as receivers of such payments. Comprehensive national health insurance legislation will surely have an impact, especially if health-care professionals other than physicians gain more power.

Nursing is a dynamic profession. The development of the nurse practitioner concept is an important example. Materials on scope of practice, standards of care, and nursing functions help to define the role nurses can play in primary care for women.[2-5] Nurses are assuming more responsibility and, consequently, are becoming more accountable. "Accountability implies duty and that a reasonable standard of care will be taken in the exercise of that duty. The nurse who has learned to meld nursing and relevant legal concepts in the nursing process will not be threatened by accountability as a measure of legal liability."[6] However, nurses should not be so complacent that they neglect to protect themselves with malpractice insurance. The rates for nurses for such insurance are reasonable, especially when purchased through the professional organization.

This chapter does not pretend to exhaust the current issues involved in women's health care. Its purpose is to bring to the reader's attention some important nursing responsibilities and to highlight areas of further study. The sources listed in the For Further Reading section address the areas of self-help, consumerism, and ethical/legal issues.

References

1. Boston Women's Health Book Collective: *Our Bodies, Ourselves*, rev ed. New York, Simon & Schuster, 1976.
2. *A Statement on the Scope of Maternal and Child Health Nursing Practice.* Kansas City, Division on Maternal and Child Health Nursing Practice, American Nurses' Association, 1980.
3. *Model for Utilization of NAACOG Standards.* Chicago, Nurses' Association of the American College of Obstetricians and Gynecologists, 1977.
4. *Standards for Obstetric, Gynecologic, and Neonatal Nursing Functions.* ed 2. Washington, DC Nurses' Association of the American College of Obstetricians and Gynecologists, 1981.
5. *The Obstetric-Gynecologic Nurse Practitioner.* Chicago, American College of Obstetricians and Gynecologists and Nurses' Association of the American College of Obstetricians and Gynecologists, 1979.
6. Murchison I, Nichols TS, Hanson R: *Legal Accountability in the Nursing Process.* St. Louis, CV Mosby, 1978, p 151.

For Further Reading

Anyan WR Jr: *Adolescent Medicine in Primary Care.* New York, Wiley, 1978.

Bates B: *A Guide to Physical Assessment,* ed 2. Philadelphia, Lippincott, 1979.

Berger K, Fields W: *Pocket Guide to Health Assessment.* Reston, Va, Reston Publishing, 1980.

Bermosk L, Porter SE: *Women's Health and Human Wholeness.* New York, Appleton-Century-Crofts, 1979.

Bernstein L, Bernstein RS, Dana RH: *Interviewing: A Guide for Health Professionals,* ed 2. New York, Appleton-Century-Crofts, 1974.

Boston Women's Health Book Collective: *Our Bodies, Ourselves,* rev ed. New York, Simon & Schuster, 1976.

Chiappa JA, Forish JJ: *The VD Book.* New York, Holt, Rinehart & Winston, 1977.

Clark AL, Affonso DD with Harris TR: *Childbearing: A Nursing Perspective,* ed 2. Philadelphia, Davis, 1979.

Cooke CW, Dworkin S: *The Ms. Guide to a Woman's Health.* New York, Anchor Books, 1979.

Davis AJ, Aroskar MA: *Ethical Dilemmas and Nursing Practice.* New York, Appleton-Century-Crofts, 1978.

DeAngelis C, Curran WJ: The legal implications of the extended roles of professional nurses. *Nursing Clinics of North America* 9: 403–409, 1974.

DeGowin EL, DeGowin RL: *Bedside Diagnostic Examination,* ed 3. New York, Macmillan, 1976.

Diagram Group: *Woman's Body: An Owner's Manual.* New York, Bantam, 1978.

Federation of Feminist Women's Health Centers. *How to Stay out of the Gynecologist's Office.* Los Angeles, Women to Women Publications, 1981.

Fogel CI, Woods, NF: *Health Care of Women a Nursing Perspective.* St. Louis, CV Mosby, 1981.

Fowkes WC Jr, Hunn VK: *Clinical Assessment for the Nurse Practitioner.* St. Louis, CV Mosby, 1973.

Gerrard B, Boniface W, Love B: *Interpersonal Skills for Health Professionals.* Reston, Va, Reston Publishing, 1980.

Gillies DA, Alyn IB: *Patient Assessment and Management by the Nurse Practitioner.* Philadelphia, Saunders, 1976.

Gollober M: Screening for cervical cancer, parts 1 and 2. *Nurse Practitioner* 4: 17–18, 20–24, 31, 1979.

Gray H: *Anatomy, Descriptive and Surgical,* 1901 ed. Philadelphia, Running Press, 1974.

Green TH Jr: *Gynecology—Essentials of Clinical Practice,* ed 3. Boston, Little, Brown, 1977.

Grissum M, Spengler C: *Womanpower and Health Care.* Boston, Little, Brown, 1976.

Hatcher RA, et al: *Contraceptive Technology 1980–1981,* ed 10. New York, Irvington, 1980.

Hawkins JW, Higgins LP: *Maternity and Gynecological Nursing: Women's Health Care.* Philadelphia, Lippincott, 1981.

Jacox AK, Norris CM: *Organizing for Independent Nursing Practice.* New York, Appleton-Century-Crofts, 1977.

Kjervik DK, Martinson IM: *Women in Stress: A Nursing Perspective.* New York: Appleton-Century-Crofts, 1979.

Lamonica EL: *The Nursing Process: A Humanistic Approach.* Menlo Park, California, Addison-Wesley, 1979.

Leininger M (ed): *Transcultural Health Care Issues and Conditions.* Philadelphia, Davis, 1976.

Leitch CJ, Tinker RV: *Primary Care.* Philadelphia, Davis, 1978.

Lytle NA (ed): *Nursing of Women in the Age of Liberation.* Dubuque, Ia, WC Brown Publishers, 1977.

MacKeith N (ed): *The New Women's Health Handbook.* London, Virago, 1978.

Marieskind HI: The women's health movement. *Nursing Dimensions* **7**: 64–67, 1979.

Marieskind HI: *Women in the Health System.* St. Louis, CV Mosby, 1980.

Martin L: *Health Care of Women.* Philadelphia, Lippincott, 1978.

McKenzie CA, Cohn SD (ed): The menopausal woman. *Issues in Health Care of Women* 1, 1978.

Murchison I, Nichols TS, Hanson R: *Legal Accountability in the Nursing Process.* St. Louis, CV Mosby, 1978.

Murray RB, Zentner JP: *Nursing Assessment & Health Promotion Through the Life Span*, ed 2. Englewood Cliffs, NJ, Prentice-Hall, 1979.

Netter FH: *The CIBA Collection of Medical Illustrations, Volume 2, Reproductive System*, rev ed. Summit, NJ, CIBA, 1965.

National Women's Health Network. Resource Guides 1, *Breast Cancer*, 2 *Hysterectomy*, 6 *DES*, 7 *Self Help.* Washington, DC, National Women's Health Network, 1980.

Novak ER, Jones GS, Jones HW Jr: *Gynecology*, ed 9. Baltimore, Williams and Wilkins, 1975.

Patient assessment: examination of the female pelvis, part 1 & 2. *American Journal of Nursing* **11, 12:** 1–26, 1–28, 1978.

Prior JA, Silberstein JS: *Physical Diagnosis*, ed 5. St. Louis, CV Mosby, 1977.

Romney SL et al: *Gynecology and Obstetrics: The Health Care of Women.* New York, McGraw-Hill, 1975.

Ruzek SK: Emergent modes of utilization: gynecological self-help. *Nursing Dimensions* **7**: 73–77, 1979.

Sandelowski M: *Women, Health, and Choice.* Englewood Cliffs, NJ, Prentice-Hall, 1981.

Shapiro HI: *The Birth Control Book.* New York, Avon Books, 1978.

Sherman JL Jr, Fields SK: *Guide to Patient Evaluation.* Flushing, NY, Medical Examination Publishing, 1974.

Sloane E: *Biology of Women.* New York, Wiley, 1980.

Stewart F, Guest F, Stewart G, et al: *My Body My Health: The Concerned Woman's Guide to Gynecology.* New York, Wiley, 1979.

Stromborg MF, Stromborg P: *Primary Care Assessment and Management Skills for Nurses: A Self-Assessment Manual.* Philadelphia, Lippincott, 1979.

Trandel-Korenchuk DM, Trandel-Korenchuk KM: How state laws recognize advanced nursing practice. *Nursing Outlook* **26:** 713–719, 1978.

Tyrer LB, Granzig WA: The new morality, ethics, and nursing. *Journal of Obstetric, Gynecologic and Neonatal Nursing* **2:** 54–55, 1973.

Widmann FK: *Goodale's Clinical Interpretation of Laboratory Tests*, ed 7. Philadelphia, Davis, 1973.

Woman's body/woman's mind, regular feature. *MS.*

Woods NF: *Human Sexuality in Health and Illness*, ed 2. St. Louis, CV Mosby, 1979.

Appendix: Protocol for Diaphragms*

1. Be completely assured that patient is a good candidate for the diaphragm. This includes adequate pelvic anatomy.

2. Conduct breast, abdominal, and pelvic exam, including Pap as indicated.

3. Adequate time for teaching is essential. Never expect the patient to be able to accomplish the initial insertion and removal by herself in the bathroom.

4. Use fitting diaphragms (not rings) for both fitting and teaching. Arcing spring, coil spring, and flat spring diaphragms should be available.

5. Be assured that patient can satisfactorily insert and remove the diaphragm herself before she leaves the clinic.

6. Follow up visit with diaphragm in place in one week.

7. Whenever patient has a vaginal infection, use cold sterilization to clean the diaphragm: soak for 30 minutes in Betadyne Scrub, not solution (Prepadyne), or in 70% rubbing alcohol.

8. Persistent back pain may indicate:
   - diaphragm is too large
   - patient is constipated
   - rim is too firm if arcing diaphragm—then a flat or coil spring should be used.

9. Informed consent must be reviewed and signed.

10. Diaphragm refit should be done after 15 lb weight gain or loss, miscarriage, abortion, baby or abdominal surgery.

*Prepared by and used with permission of Mary Fahey, RN, Gyn NP; Mary Kurien, RN, C, MS, Gyn NP; Diane Roberto, RN, C, Gyn NP; J Lynn Stanley, RN, C, ANP; Carol Frankinburger, RN, C, ANP, 1981 of the Women's Health Clinic, Student Health Services, University of Connecticut, Storrs, Connecticut.

Reference for fitting diaphragms

Bradbury B: "Preventing the diaphragm baby syndrome": a matter of technique, teaching and time. *Journal of Obstetric, Gynecologic and Neonatal Nursing* **4:** 25–32, 1975.

Index